American Cancer Society's Guide to

Pain Control

American Cancer Society's Guide to

Pain Control

Understanding and Managing Cancer Pain

Revised Edition

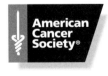

From the Experts at the
American Cancer Society

Published by
American Cancer Society
Health Promotions
1599 Clifton Road NE
Atlanta, Georgia 30329, USA

Printed in the United States of America
Cover designed by Jill Dible

5 4 3 2 1   04 05 06 07 08

Library of Congress Cataloging-in-Publication Data

American Cancer Society's guide to pain control : understanding and managing cancer pain.— Rev. ed.
    p. cm.
Previous ed. has subtitle: Powerful methods to overcome cancer pain.
Includes bibliographical references and index.
  ISBN 0-944235-52-2 (pbk. : alk. paper)
 1. Cancer pain. 2. cancer pain—Treatment. I. Title: Guide to pain control. II. American Cancer Society.

  RC262.A645 2004
  616'.0472—dc22
                                2003025526

Brief Contents

EDITOR
Amy Brittain

MANAGING EDITOR
Gianna Marsella, MA

BOOK PUBLISHING MANAGER
Candace Magee

DIRECTOR, PUBLISHING
Diane Scott-Lichter, MA

DIRECT CHANNELS
MANAGING DIRECTOR
Chuck Westbrook

EDITORIAL REVIEW
Terri Ades, MS, APRN-BC, AOCN
Director of Cancer Information
American Cancer Society
Atlanta, Georgia

Betty R. Ferrell, PhD, FAAN
Research Scientist
City of Hope National Medical Center
Duarte, California

A Note to the Reader

The information contained in this book is not intended as medical advice and should not be relied upon as a substitute for talking with your doctor. This information may not address all possible actions, precautions, side effects, or interactions. All matters regarding your health require the supervision of a medical doctor who is familiar with your medical needs. For more information, contact your American Cancer Society at 800-ACS-2345 or http://www.cancer.org.

Contents

Foreword

by Betty R. Ferrell, PhD, FAAN, Research Scientist
City of Hope National Medical Center, Duarte, California

PAIN HAS THE POTENTIAL TO NEGATIVELY AFFECT physical, psychological, social, sexual, and spiritual well-being, as well as upset family members and caregivers. Providing all available pain-relief methods to people with cancer is not only essential for preserving quality of life, it is critical to successful cancer treatment. Patients are better able to tolerate cancer treatment when their pain is alleviated.

The American Cancer Society is dedicated to diminishing suffering from cancer and has focused major efforts—including the publication of the first and revised editions of this book—toward addressing the critical issue of pain management and enhancing quality of life for people facing cancer.

Advances in Understanding Pain

Major advances in cancer prevention, early detection, diagnosis, and treatment have been mirrored by major advances in the understanding and treatment of cancer pain. In 1994, the federal government issued guidelines for the treatment of cancer pain. These initial guidelines, published by the Agency for Health Care Policy and Research, have been reinforced and elaborated upon through major documents from the National Cancer Institute, professional organizations, and consumer groups. All of these groups have consistently agreed that pain negatively affects quality of life—and that, unfortunately, pain is often undertreated.

Partnering to Manage Pain

The successful management of pain requires a partnership between patients and health care professionals. People with cancer and caregivers who are informed about cancer pain will better understand the importance of expressing pain, overcoming fears of addiction and tolerance, exploring appropriate nondrug methods of pain relief, and expecting that all means available are used to provide optimal pain relief. Cancer care professionals can help improve quality of life for people in pain by understanding how to overcome social and cultural barriers, balance side effects of pain-control methods, and assess and treat pain.

The Role of this Book in Pain Control

The *American Cancer Society's Guide to Pain Control* was first published in 2001 to inform patients and their families about cancer pain, how to manage it, and how to obtain the best pain-control care possible. The revised edition of this comprehensive resource for patients, families, and health care professionals reflects updated developments in pain control, with an increased focus on practical information for people with cancer. It is essential reading for people with cancer and their family members. This book explains how to take control of cancer pain and how to obtain emotional and social support, and emphasizes that pain can usually be alleviated.

Everyone Has a Right to Pain Relief

Research and advances in clinical practice in the last decade have provided strong evidence that cancer pain is not a necessary part of having cancer, and the majority of people with cancer should expect to experience relief from cancer pain. More and more people are living with cancer, and this population must be able to participate in work, family, and enjoyable activities without being hindered or debilitated by pain. Quality of life must also be preserved for special populations, such as infants and children, the elderly, patients with a history of substance abuse, patients from diverse cultures, and those who are critically ill.

Continuous efforts are being made in the oncology field to better inform health care professionals about the importance of preventing, assessing, and managing pain. Health care professionals should not only strive to prevent pain before it occurs, but continue to learn more about the origins of pain and shape state-of-the-art treatments to treat it. The cooperation between patients and medical professionals is as critical as ever; pain relief can only be achieved through the effective description and assessment of pain.

As our knowledge about cancer pain and how to manage it grow, so do the range of powerful pain-prevention and pain-relief resources at our disposal, including medications, nondrug methods, and complementary therapies. All people with cancer should expect high-quality treatment and care, including a personally tailored pain-relief plan. Pain relief is a basic right and is the foundation for coping with a diagnosis of cancer. Effective pain relief enables patients to focus their energies on fighting cancer and regaining control of their lives.

Introduction

ALTHOUGH PAIN IS ONE OF THE MOST FEARED complications of cancer, many people with cancer do not experience cancer-related pain. In most cases pain can be reduced so a person with cancer can continue most daily activities. Approximately nine out of ten people who have cancer-related pain can get effective pain relief.

Today, many different kinds of medicines and other methods can help relieve pain. With effective pain management, people with cancer pain are free to sleep and eat, enjoy the company of family and friends, and continue with work, hobbies, and other pleasurable activities.

The Impact of Cancer Pain

In general, about two out of every three people with cancer experience pain sometime during their cancer experience. Although cancer pain is often thought of as a crisis that emerges in advanced stages of disease, it may occur at any stage and may be caused by many factors—cancer itself, treatments, or factors unrelated to cancer.

Pain can have a significant impact on both physical and emotional aspects of life. It can cause suffering and reduce physical and social activity, appetite, and sleep. It can weaken the body and make it difficult to follow through with scheduled treatments. Uncontrolled pain negatively affects quality of life, preventing people from working productively, enjoying recreation, or taking pleasure in their usual roles in the family and society.

The psychological effects of cancer pain can also be devastating. An inability to meet financial, employment, and interpersonal demands can create a heavy burden. People with cancer may lose hope when pain occurs because they think pain signals the progression of disease. Chronic, severe, or unrelieved pain can lead to depression, and depression or anxiety can lower a person's tolerance for pain and make the pain feel even worse.

Cancer Pain Is Undertreated

The inadequate treatment of cancer pain causes needless suffering. Although a variety of treatment methods exist to relieve cancer pain, research shows that it is still undertreated.

Even though treatments exist that can significantly reduce cancer pain and improve the quality of life of patients and their families, enormous barriers persist that can prevent these treatments from being adequately and appropriately applied. Patients' and health professionals' lack of knowledge about the appropriate use of treatments is a major barrier. Myths and misconceptions about pain, addiction, and tolerance may make patients reluctant to ask for or use pain medication and may make health professionals reluctant to prescribe pain medications. Health care professionals often lack knowledge about how to assess pain (that is, understand if the patient is having pain, and if so, how much pain, what type of pain, and its location or cause) and adequately treat pain. Fear of disciplinary action by licensing boards and criminal prosecution by drug enforcement agencies also hinders professionals from prescribing appropriate medicines and/or doses to relieve pain.

Pain control is still considered a secondary issue rather than a central element of appropriate cancer care. Until recently, hospitals and health care systems did not have practice standards for pain control (see *Appendix B* on page 201 for more information about guidelines for pain management). Health insurance companies do not adequately reimburse for pain medications, and this restricts patients' access to needed pain control. Further, because of societal and cultural barriers, patients often do not feel comfortable raising concerns about cancer pain. These barriers also inhibit doctors and nurses from appropriately and adequately prescribing pain medications and deter patients from using them.

Methods of Pain Control

Cancer pain can be treated in a variety of ways. One of the most effective methods of pain control is the use of medicines, or drug therapy. Nondrug therapies may also help manage pain, including applying heat or cold, massage, transcutaneous electrical nerve stimulation (TENS), exercise, immobilization (e.g., bracing a joint), nerve blocks and nervous system surgery, and acupuncture.

Pain relief can also be achieved by reducing a person's reaction to pain. People can learn skills such as relaxation, imagery, meditation, distraction, biofeedback, hypnosis, and other techniques to increase their ability to cope with pain and remain as active as possible. These complementary nondrug methods can also help people cope with the emotional and psychological impact of pain on their quality of life and well-being, both of which can be significantly affected by pain.

What You Can Do

The first step in pain control is to identify and express the pain. If your doctor does not bring up the subject of pain, it is up to you to make your pain known. The cornerstone of effective pain management is a thorough pain assessment. What you tell your health care team about your pain and how you describe your pain help form the pain assessment. You can help by describing your experience of pain in as much detail as possible. Only you can describe the nature of your pain to your health care team, including:

- the location
- what it feels like
- how long it lasts
- when it started
- the intensity or how severe it is
- what makes it better and what makes it worse

Recording and reporting the effects of your pain and how it impacts your ability to function every day will also help with the evaluation. Your doctor will use your information along with a detailed history, physical examination, psychosocial assessment, and the results of any diagnostic studies to determine the treatment options that are best for you.

How to Use This Book

The *American Cancer Society's Guide to Pain Control* is a comprehensive guide that will help you understand the complex issues involved in dealing with cancer pain. The goal of this book is to help people affected by cancer pain:

- learn about pain
- overcome the barriers to pain treatment
- communicate with members of the health care team, including describing pain accurately
- manage pain and related side effects
- cope with the related emotional and social concerns
- find helpful resources in the community and across the country

This book will walk you through the important issues and details related to pain control, from diagnosis throughout your cancer experience. You'll discover how to achieve acceptable pain control and how to understand the optimal balance between pain relief and side effects of pain medication. As you read, you'll learn about how cancer pain and its treatment affect your body, your emotions, your relationships with others, and your life in general. We encourage you to evaluate the information here and talk with your health care team to determine how best to treat your pain. Remember that you have a right to receive appropriate treatment for pain control.

About the American Cancer Society

Represented in more than 3,400 communities throughout the country and Puerto Rico, the American Cancer Society is a nonprofit health organization dedicated to eliminating cancer as a major health problem. This book is just one example of the many ways the American Cancer Society seeks to fulfill its mission: to save lives and diminish suffering from cancer through research, education, advocacy, and service.

The Society is the largest private source of cancer research dollars in the U.S. Approximately two million Americans volunteer their time to the Society to work to conquer cancer. To contact the American Cancer Society, call 800-ACS-2345 or visit our web site at http://www.cancer.org.

Acknowledgments

Many people helped shape this edition of the *American Cancer Society's Guide to Pain Control* by providing us with valuable feedback on the first edition of this text:

Terri Ades, MS, APRN-BC, AOCN; Claudia Barnes, RN, BSN, CHPN; Debbie Bruins; Melinda Burns; Patrick J. Coyne, MSN, APRN, BC-PCM; Sherryll Crutcher; June Dahl, PhD; Doreen Donahue, OSW-C; Pat Dooley, RNC, BSN, MHSA; Wendy J. Evans, RN, MSN, AOCN; Betty R. Ferrell, PhD, FAAN; Walter B. Forman, MD, FACP, CMD; Michele E. Gaguski, MSN, RN, AOCN, APN-C; Lisa L. Hansen; Dionetta M. Hudzinski, RN, MN; Pat Kennedy, RN, CHPN; Mary Pat Lynch, CRNP, MSN, AOCN; Mary E. Murphy, RN, MS, AOCN, CHPN; Judith Paice, PhD, RN; Diana Peirce, RN, CHPN; Peg Rummel, RN, BSN, MHA, OCN; Linda Schickedanz, RN, MSN; Judy Schnack, MSN, RN, FNP; Susan Ann Small, RN; Karen Stevenson, RN, MS; Lucien Winegar; Donna Zhukovsky, MD, FACP.

We thank them for the time, energy, and expertise they generously dedicated to this project. We are also especially grateful to Mary Bennett for helping us locate individuals willing to review our text.

CHAPTER 1

Understanding Cancer Pain

A fter she was first diagnosed, Melissa was afraid that she would have pain. Actually, she thought cancer and pain went hand in hand. She had pain with her surgery, but it was well controlled and soon went away. After surgery, she feared having more pain even though her cancer had been removed. She could not block the memories of her father dying in pain from his cancer. She expected to have pain just like him. She has been without any evidence of disease for nine years. And she has no pain.

ONE OF THE FIRST STEPS IN MANAGING YOUR PAIN is learning about it. Having cancer does not always mean being in pain. If pain does occur, there are many ways to relieve or reduce it. Relieving pain makes you more comfortable, while untreated pain puts your body under additional stress. New studies show that improved pain control increases survival and quality of life. This chapter will discuss the nature of pain and give you the language you need to communicate with your health care team about your pain.

What Is Cancer?

Before exploring types of cancer pain and how to relieve them, we'll briefly explore cancer itself—what it is and how it forms.

Cancer is not just one disease; it's as many as 100 different diseases with one thing in common—the growth and spread of abnormal cells because of gene mutations (structural or chemical changes within genes that change the way cells function and grow).

Normal cells grow, divide, and die in an orderly fashion. During the early years of a person's life, normal cells divide more rapidly until the person becomes an adult. After that, normal cells of most tissues divide only to replace worn-out or dying cells and to repair injuries.

Some cells, however, continue to grow and divide and may also spread to other parts of the body. These abnormal cells accumulate and form a tumor. Malignant tumors are lumps that have the potential to spread and may invade and destroy normal tissue. If cells break away from a cancerous tumor, they can travel to other areas of the body. There, they may settle and form "colony" tumors, continuing to grow. The spread of a tumor to a new site is called metastasis.

What Is Pain?

Pain is a sensation that hurts. It is a warning signal that something is wrong in our bodies. A variety of factors may cause pain in people with cancer; however, not all people with cancer will experience pain. When pain does occur, the experience may range from mild discomfort to severe agony. While some people experience pain for only a short period of time, others may cope with chronic pain for months, seriously impacting their ability to do the things they enjoy.

Pain has two main components: a sensory component and a reactive component. The sensory component involves the transmission, or sending of, the pain signal from the injured part of the body to the spinal cord and brain. When the pain signal is received, the brain then sends a message to the person that he or she is having pain. The reactive component refers to how the person reacts to the pain. Each person's reaction to pain depends upon his or her pain threshold (the intensity of the stimulus a person considers painful) and pain tolerance (how intense or how long the pain stimulus can persist before the person experiences the pain). People can have differences in their pain thresholds and pain tolerances.

Types of Pain

The type of pain a person experiences depends on its source. Cancer-related pain occurs because of something related to the cancer, either the disease or the treatment of it. Most cancer pain is caused by the cancer itself, but pain can also occur because of the side effects of cancer treatment—such as radiation therapy, chemotherapy, and surgery. People with cancer may also have pain that is not related to cancer.

Pain can be acute, chronic, or breakthrough, depending on how long the pain is present and when it occurs. It can also be categorized as nociceptive or neuropathic pain, medical terms that sometimes suggest the cause of the pain. We'll explore each of these types of pain in this chapter.

Acute Pain

Acute pain is usually severe, begins suddenly, and lasts a relatively short time. It is often a signal that body tissue is being injured in some way, and acute pain generally disappears when the injury heals.

Acute pain may be caused by surgery, a burn, a cut, or a needle stick, for example. Some cancer treatment or treatment side effects can also cause acute pain; for example, surgery to remove a tumor, sores in the mouth from chemotherapy, or inflammation of the rectal area after radiation treatment for prostate cancer. A person in acute pain may have symptoms that reflect they are in pain, such as an increase in blood pressure and a rapid heartbeat. The symptoms of acute pain can be more severe than those of other types of pain. Acute pain that lasts for more than a few weeks becomes chronic pain.

Chronic Pain

Chronic pain, which can range from mild to severe, may be ongoing and may last for several months. It can result from the cancer itself or from treatment. The most common type of pain in people with cancer is bone pain caused by cancer metastasizing to the bone. Another type of chronic pain is caused by a tumor pressing on organs or nerves. After chronic pain has been present for a while, the body adjusts to it and the physical intensity will be lessened, but a person's ability to function and continue activities can still be severely impacted. Having to cope with chronic pain on a daily basis can lead to irritability, disturbed sleep, reduced appetite, difficulty concentrating, and changes in mood, personality, lifestyle, and ability to function. Because chronic pain can make even the simplest tasks and daily activities uncomfortable or impossible, people in chronic pain may have feelings of hopelessness and depression—negative thoughts and emotions that can make pain feel worse. To reduce overall suffering, chronic pain should be treated as quickly as possible.

Breakthrough Pain

Many people with chronic cancer pain have two types of pain: persistent (continuous) pain and breakthrough (incident) pain. Persistent pain is present for long periods of time—in most cases, all day long. Breakthrough pain is a brief and often severe flare of pain that occurs even though a person may be taking pain medicine regularly for persistent pain. It's called breakthrough pain because it is pain that "breaks through" a regular pain medicine schedule. It is not unusual for people with persistent pain to experience episodes of breakthrough pain.

Breakthrough pain may be different for each person and is often unpredictable. It typically comes on quickly, lasts only a few minutes or as long as an hour, and feels much like persistent pain except that it is more severe. Breakthrough pain can be caused by the cancer itself or may be related to the treatment of cancer. Some people have breakthrough pain during a certain activity, like walking or dressing. For others, breakthrough pain occurs unexpectedly and has no clear cause.

In the example below, the individual has persistent pain and is regularly taking pain medication. However, this patient has two episodes of breakthrough pain, at 1 p.m. and at 7 p.m. He will need a medication for the breakthrough pain that acts quickly to relieve this pain.

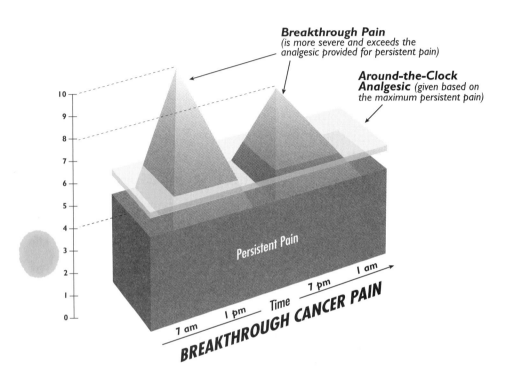

Nociceptive Pain

Nociceptive pain involves damage to body tissue. When a person's body tissue is injured, pain receptors (thousands of nerve endings located throughout the body, called nociceptors) are activated, sending a signal to the spinal cord and brain that is interpreted as pain. When a person feels pain from cancer that has spread to muscle, bone, organs, and joints, the pain is called nociceptive pain. Nociceptive pain may be acute or chronic. The source of nociceptive pain is easier to locate than the source of neuropathic pain.

Neuropathic Pain

Neuropathic pain is caused by injury to, or compression of, some part of the nervous system, which includes the peripheral nerves and the central nervous system. It can result from either the cancer itself or from treatment. People often describe neuropathic pain as severe burning, sharp, tingling, or shooting pain. Neuropathic pain can also cause a loss of feeling in an area of the body or a feeling of extreme tenderness, making the lightest touch painful.

An example of neuropathic pain is post-mastectomy syndrome. Following surgery to remove a breast, a person will have some post-operative pain. After that pain subsides, the person will be able to return to normal activities. Some time later, pain may return to the original painful area without a clear cause. This pain may be described as a "strange" burning, pressure, shooting, stabbing, or knifelike sensation, or as pain or numbness. This pain is due to damage to nerves in the breast area and is referred to as post-mastectomy syndrome.

Factors that Influence Pain

Pain thresholds and pain tolerances differ from person to person, but how pain is perceived depends on how it is processed by a person through feelings, thoughts, and memories of pain. Past experiences with pain or the cause of the pain can influence a person's reaction to a new pain. For example, people who have seen the death of a friend or family member who was in pain may be terrified at the thought of pain because they associate pain with death. For a professional baseball pitcher, pain resulting from a sprained ankle may perhaps be minimized or ignored. He knows his life is not in danger from the cause of pain and he may be receiving significant reward for ignoring the pain and continuing to play.

Some people feel hopeless or helpless when in pain. Others may feel alone, embarrassed, inadequate, angry, frightened, or frantic. These strong emotions can have a significant effect on how people experience pain and how they cope with it. Rest, understanding, support, analgesics (medicines to relieve pain), and reducing anxiety can raise the pain threshold. However, other factors—such as fatigue, depression, or anxiety—can lower the pain threshold and make the pain feel worse. Dealing with these factors and their underlying causes is important in reducing pain (see chapter 2 for information about coping with feelings related to cancer and cancer pain).

Causes of Pain

Pain may be caused by various factors or combinations of factors, including diagnostic procedures, treatment, cancer itself, or other reasons. Pain is not inevitable; talk to your health care team about a pain-relief plan that's right for you and your situation. Chapters 5 through 7 provide more information about pain-relief options.

Diagnostic Procedures

In order to make an accurate cancer diagnosis and to determine the extent of the cancer, your health care team needs to do some diagnostic procedures. Some of these procedures may cause temporary pain and discomfort, lasting only for the duration of the test or for a day or two afterwards. More invasive procedures may cause pain that lasts several days or longer. In the following sections we will outline some of the most common diagnostic procedures that may cause pain or discomfort, as well as appropriate preventive or coping measures, so you know what to expect and can better cope with potential pain. Talk to your

About Fatigue

What to look for:
- having no energy
- sleeping more
- not wanting to do normal activities
- paying less attention to personal appearance
- feeling tired even after sleeping
- having trouble concentrating

What to do:
- Schedule necessary activities throughout the day rather than all at once; light activity or regular exercise may be helpful.
- Plan brief rest periods to conserve energy for important things.
- Get enough rest and sleep.
- Eat a nutritious diet and drink plenty of liquids.
- Let others help you with meals, housework, or errands.

Do not:
- force yourself to do more than you can manage
- think that you are just being "lazy"

Call your doctor or nurse if:
- you are too tired to get out of bed for more than a 24-hour period
- you become confused
- the fatigue becomes progressively worse
- you have severe or frequent dizziness
- you feel out of breath

health care team about your situation and how you might prevent or alleviate pain from diagnostic procedures.

Biopsy

A biopsy is the removal of a sample of tissue that is examined to determine whether cancer cells are present. A type of device is used to remove the tissue, often a sterile knife or needle. Some biopsies can be done on an outpatient basis while others may require a hospital stay. A needle biopsy may cause temporary discomfort and pain at the site of insertion. A more invasive procedure such as a surgical biopsy may involve postoperative pain and discomfort.

Bone Marrow Aspiration and Biopsy

A bone marrow aspiration involves removing a small amount of bone marrow, the soft material inside bones where blood cells are formed. During a bone marrow biopsy, a small cylindrical piece of bone and bone marrow (about $\frac{1}{16}$ inch in diameter and $\frac{1}{2}$ inch long) is removed. A local anesthetic is given before the needle is inserted into the skin. Often, a sharp jolt and a sensation of intense pressure can be felt when the marrow is withdrawn. The puncture site may also be bruised and tender for a few days.

Endoscopy

This is a medical procedure for viewing the interior of the body through a hollow, tube-like instrument. Some endoscopes not only allow the doctor to see inside the body, they can also be used for surgery. Small instruments operated through the hollow endoscope are used to remove biopsy specimens (small pieces of tissue used for laboratory tests) or even to remove or destroy a tumor. Because there is sometimes discomfort during an endoscopy, anesthesia or sedatives may be used. The procedure can be performed on an outpatient basis, in a doctor's office, or it may require a hospital stay. The recovery time varies depending upon the method used.

Endometrial Biopsy

An endometrial biopsy is an office procedure in which a sample of endometrial tissue is removed by a small instrument inserted into the uterus through the cervix. The degree and duration of pain vary, but the discomfort is similar to severe menstrual cramps and can be helped by taking a nonsteroidal anti-inflammatory drug such as ibuprofen an hour before the procedure.

Lumbar Puncture (Spinal Tap)

A lumbar puncture is a test in which a needle is placed in the lower back into the spinal canal, to give medicine into the central nervous system through the spinal fluid or to obtain a small sample of cerebrospinal fluid, which is examined under a microscope to determine if cancer cells are present. Patients may develop painful and severe headaches after this procedure. The pain, which feels worse when standing up, can last from a few hours to several days. The headache can usually be treated with bed rest and medication.

Cancer Treatment

There are many different ways to treat cancer, but the main types of treatment are surgery, chemotherapy, and radiation. Because each treatment is different and the appropriate treatment for each person's situation depends on the person's overall health, type of cancer, and stage of disease, it is difficult to predict who will experience pain from a particular treatment.

As much fear as pain may instill in people, there is no need to suffer through pain without some kind of help. Learning to talk to your doctor, nurse, or someone on your health care team about pain and pain-relief needs can bring the relief that most people with cancer-related pain need and that all of them deserve. Living with pain does not need to be a standard aspect of undergoing cancer treatment.

Surgery

Surgery is the oldest form of treatment for cancer and offers the greatest chance of cure for many types of cancer. About 60 percent of people with cancer will have some type of surgery. The pain experienced by people after surgery is generally of two types:

1. Acute, temporary pain—focused around the area of incision (surgical cutting), which is related to the healing and recovery process.
2. Chronic or long-term pain—resulting from injury to nerves, muscles, organs, or other tissue in the area where cancerous tumors and other tissue may have been removed.

After surgery, a person may feel tired, sore, and generally uncomfortable until the incision is fully healed and moving around is easier. The pain associated with surgery is common, will go away after several days, and can be controlled. However, some people may experience chronic pain resulting from damage to the body or nerves during surgery. Surgery can also result in some painful side effects such as lymphedema or phantom limb pain, both of which can occur after the removal of an appendage or body part. We will explore nerve pain, lymphedema, and phantom limb pain here.

NERVE PAIN FROM SURGICAL PROCEDURES

Some surgical procedures can cause injury to underlying nerves, which can lead to chronic pain for some people. This kind of pain can develop weeks or months after surgery and is usually located at the incision site. Pain resulting from nerve damage is much more difficult to treat than pain from a surgical incision. Talk with your health care team about how to address and cope with nerve pain.

LYMPHEDEMA

Mastectomy, or removal of the breast, can include the removal of lymph nodes and vessels under the arm. After lymph nodes are removed, if the remaining lymph vessels cannot remove enough lymph fluid in the breast and underarm area, the excess fluid builds up and causes painful swelling, or lymphedema. Lymphedema can range from mild to severe and can occur soon after surgery or many months or even years later.

Lymphedema should be treated by a physical therapist or other health care professional who has had special training in lymphedema care. One method of treatment for lymphedema, often called Complex Decongestive Therapy (CDT), consists of skin care, massage, special bandaging, exercise, and fitting for a compression sleeve.

PHANTOM LIMB PAIN

After a body part is removed during surgery, such as in a mastectomy or amputation, a person may still feel pain or other unpleasant sensations such as burning or tingling that seem as if they are coming from the absent limb or breast. Phantom limb pain is not only physically uncomfortable, it can cause emotional anxiety as well. No single pain-relief method will control phantom limb pain in all patients all the time, but a variety of treatments may be used to effectively treat it, including pain medication, physical therapy, and nerve stimulation (see chapters 5 through 7 for more information about pain-relief options).

Chemotherapy

Chemotherapy is the use of anticancer medicines to kill cancer cells. Some people who take chemotherapy experience no painful side effects, but others do.

Some people experience mild pain from the constant use of needles if chemotherapy is given by needle in the vein, especially when several cycles of chemotherapy are given over several months' time. Devices are available that can help minimize the number of times needles have to be used to deliver the drugs used in chemotherapy. If some chemotherapy medicines are allowed to leak out of the vein, they can cause mild to severe tissue damage and pain. The possibility is decreased when a highly skilled medical professional administers the medication.

One of the most common and painful side effects of chemotherapy is inflammation or sores of the mouth, throat, esophagus, or tongue, which can make swallowing, eating, and talking difficult. These side effects can lead to bleeding, painful ulceration, and infection and are most often treated with pain medication and topical anesthetics (numbing medication) which can be applied directly to the sores.

Another possible side effect of some chemotherapy medicines is irritation or damage involving the nerves that send sensations from the hands, fingers, feet, and toes. This can lead to pain, tingling sensations, numbness, and sometimes loss of function in hands, fingers, feet, and toes.

Radiation Therapy

Radiation therapy is another commonly used treatment for cancer. An estimated 50 to 60 percent of all people with cancer receive radiation at some point during their cancer treatment. Radiation therapy involves focusing an invisible ray or beam on a region of the body where the cancer is located (in some situations, a small pellet containing a radioactive substance may be put into a tumor) to decrease the size of tumors and relieve symptoms.

Some of the side effects of radiation treatment can cause pain and discomfort. For example, skin exposed to radiation treatment may peel or become irritated. These skin changes can be quite painful and can put a person at risk for infection. Appropriate skin care measures are used to minimize these skin effects. Radiation therapy can cause damage to any tissue in the field of the radiation, though great care is taken in treatment planning to avoid tissue damage to bones, nerves, and organs, for example. Damage to these parts of the body may cause pain. If the spinal cord is in the radiation field and receives too much radiation, pain will occur in various parts of the body, depending on the level of damage.

The mucous membranes, such as the lining of the mouth, are also sensitive to radiation. Some mouth cancers may require high doses of radiation. A dry mouth, change in taste, and inflammation of the lining of the mouth may result from radiation to the head and neck area and may make it difficult to eat. Taking pain medications or using topical anesthetics to numb the mouth before meals may make it easier to eat. If the pain and irritation become too severe, some people may need to have a feeding tube inserted into their stomach so they can receive adequate nutrition.

Tumor-Related Pain

Tumor-related pain can affect many different parts of the body. The type and degree of pain will vary with size and location of the tumor. When pain is caused by a tumor, cancer treatments (surgery, chemotherapy, or radiation therapy) are used to reduce the tumor size and relieve pain. Other pain-control measures, such as pain medications, are also used along with the cancer treatment to treat the pain.

Gastrointestinal (GI) Obstruction

Pain in the abdomen can be the result of a tumor blocking, or obstructing, the stomach, small intestines, or colon. This can cause diarrhea, constipation, abdominal swelling, cramping, nausea, or vomiting. GI obstruction sometimes occurs with colorectal or ovarian cancer; however, it can also occur from any tumor that begins in or spreads to the abdomen. Different types of abdominal pain can occur with tumors in different parts of the abdomen.

Intracranial Pressure/Metastases of the Skull

Tumors within any part of the brain may cause increased pressure within the skull, sometimes referred to as intracranial pressure. Increased pressure within the skull may cause headaches, nausea, vomiting, or blurred vision. More than half of people with brain tumors experience headaches involving steady, aching, dull pain. Cancer that has spread, or metastasized, to the base of the skull may cause face, neck, or shoulder pain, headaches, or pain when moving the head. Head and neck pain can be a sign of spinal cord compression from a tumor, one of the most serious complications of bone metastasis. In this condition, pressure on the spinal cord is caused by metastases extending from the spinal bones or by collapse of the spinal bones, which can cause pain, numbness, or paralysis. Spinal cord compression can also occur when other cancers spread to the spine, as in prostate cancer.

Bone Pain

Cancer that has spread to the bone is one of the most frequent causes of pain in people with cancer and can also cause fractures, hypercalcemia (high blood calcium levels due to the release of calcium from damaged bones), spinal cord compression, as well as other symptoms and complications that negatively affect a person's quality of life. Bone pain is often the earliest sign of bone metastasis, but it is not always the only symptom. The pain often comes and goes at first, tends to be worse at night, and may be relieved by movement. Later on, it becomes a constant dull ache and may be worse during activity. Fractures (broken bones) due to bone metastasis can cause severe pain and, because they heal slowly if at all, can severely limit mobility.

Nerve Pain

Nerve damage can cause disturbing and sometimes debilitating pain. It causes sensations such as tingling, burning, pressing, squeezing, pinching, itching, and numbness. Nerve pain is usually constant and steady and is sometimes accompanied by shooting or jolting pain similar to a seizure or convulsion. Nerve damage can be accompanied by bladder or bowel weakness, motor or reflex problems, or impaired senses such as poor taste or smell. Some patients also suffer from what is known as evoked pain, an unpleasant, abnormal sensation in which a patient has unusual pain sensitivity from something as ordinary as touch.

Pain Due to Other Causes

Having cancer does not make a person immune to other illnesses. Pain can occur because of illnesses not related to cancer, including stomach or digestion problems, back strain, migraine headaches, shingles, arthritis, inflammation and infection, and injuries.

Pain Caused by Immobility

Pain from immobility can occur when a person (for any of a variety of medical reasons, including cancer and treatment) is too fatigued to exercise or move around normally. Difficulty moving is a problem characterized by general weakness and problems with walking, for example, after a person spends a lot of time in bed. A lack of movement results in weakened muscles and problems such as poor or no appetite, constipation, increased fatigue, skin sores, difficulty breathing, stiff joints, and mental changes.

Help Is on the Way

Pain is not an inevitable result of cancer. When it does occur, effective treatments are available. Doctors and other medical professionals can help you reduce or eliminate pain using relatively simple and proven measures tailored to the cause of your pain. Pain can usually be reduced to manageable levels. Chapter 4 will help you explain your pain to your health care providers so that you can get the most effective relief possible. The chapters that follow will help you cope with the emotional and social impact of cancer pain, understand methods of pain relief, and manage medication side effects.

CHAPTER 2

Coping with the Emotional and Social Impact of Cancer Pain

here is a fear that goes through you when you are told you have cancer. It's so hard in the beginning to think about anything but your diagnosis. It's the first thing you think about every morning. I want people diagnosed with cancer to know it does get better. Talking about your cancer helps you deal with all of the new emotions you are feeling. Remember that it's normal to get upset."

— Delores, a cancer survivor

PAIN IS ONE OF THE MOST IMPORTANT FACTORS affecting the lives of people with cancer. Reducing or eliminating cancer-related pain may result in fewer emotional and psychological challenges, improved outlook and mood, greater optimism about the future, and better ability to cope with cancer and cancer treatment.

Pain's Impact on Quality of Life

Pain is not a purely physical experience. It can profoundly affect your emotional, social, and spiritual well-being. Pain can interfere with your normal daily activities and diminish your enjoyment of everyday pleasures, prevent relaxation and sleep, and increase anxiety, stress, and fatigue. It can also make people withdraw from others; individuals with continuous mild or moderate pain often report that their social activities decrease and that they have less contact with friends and family. In other words, pain impairs your ability to do the things you want to do—it negatively affects your quality of life.

When the source of pain is cancer, pain's psychological, or mental, impact is often magnified. Physical pain can intensify emotions evoked by a diagnosis of cancer, such as fear, anxiety, worry, and depression. Pain may cause feelings of helplessness, depression, isolation, anger, and even guilt. Some people may believe their pain is punishment for something they've done or may feel guilty that they depend on friends or family when they are in pain.

What "Quality of Life" Means

Controlling pain can improve your quality of life immeasurably. But exactly what is meant by the term "quality of life"? Researchers have identified four key components that constitute quality of life:

- physical well-being, which includes things like strength, mobility, and fatigue
- psychological well-being, which includes feelings like happiness, sadness, anxiety, and fear
- interpersonal well-being, which includes relationships with family, friends, and caregivers
- spiritual well-being, which includes the meaning of suffering and the purpose of life

Measuring Quality of Life

Some of the factors that determine quality of life can be easily measured, including strength and functional abilities like walking, sleeping, and eating independently, as well as depression, anxiety, and the quality of relationships with friends and loved ones.

Only you know the amount or type of pain you feel and how it affects your daily life. You are the best judge of your pain. Research has shown that self-reporting pain is a more accurate gauge than observations from caregivers (family members or friends who help and support you during your cancer treatment) or medical personnel. Make sure your caregivers and health care team rely on your description of pain.

Common Feelings about Cancer and Cancer Pain

People cope with cancer in different ways. Most people initially feel tremendous emotional upheaval after being diagnosed with cancer. They may experience many upsetting feelings, such as disbelief, shock, fear, and anger.

Over time, most people come to terms with the reality of living with a diagnosis of cancer. After the initial shock of diagnosis and the beginning of treatment, most people find that they are able to continue much of their normal lives. They learn to adapt and continue with work, entertainment, and social relationships. Many people say that being diagnosed with cancer gave them an opportunity to reevaluate their lives and discover strengths and abilities they did not know they had. Of course, there are times when it is difficult to find strength and the situation may feel overwhelming.

Factors that Affect Feelings about Pain

Your mental outlook has a big impact on how you perceive and cope with pain. People with cancer who are depressed or anxious typically report feeling more pain than those who are calm and optimistic. Those whose daily activities are impaired by cancer and its treatment and who rely on caregivers for help also report more pain than those who are able to be self-sufficient.

Feelings and attitudes about pain may also be influenced by culture, age, and gender (see chapter 9 for more information). In some cultures, talking about pain is not encouraged and is considered "complaining." Patients from such cultures may suffer in silence even when pain relief is available. In other cultural groups, people in pain may be more vocal about their pain and insist on relief. Men and women also often differ in expressing pain-relief needs. Men are often raised to be "tough" and remain silent about pain. In general, women are more likely to acknowledge pain and ask for help. Age affects communication about pain as well; older people are less likely than younger people to talk about their pain.

Individual Reactions to Pain

Predicting how any one individual will cope with cancer pain is difficult. Everyone reacts differently. Some people may be able to carry on normal activities even while in moderate pain. Others may be incapacitated by the same level of pain. This doesn't mean that one person is tougher than another, only that there is a wide variation in the way people react to and deal with pain.

Functional limitations such as difficulty walking, eating, or sleeping, or being unable to take care of oneself may affect one person's outlook on life differently than it affects another. People whose pain keeps them from moving about comfortably may experience strong emotional reactions, such as hopelessness. Yet the same restrictions may cause minimal distress for people who are comfortable relying on others for help. One person may benefit most from pain treatment that allows more mobility, while another may be satisfied with a pain level that permits better sleep.

The degree of an individual's psychological distress in the face of pain depends on many factors, including social support, coping ability, and personality. Pain relief usually helps people cope more effectively with stress and deal with the reality of cancer and its implications.

A person's spirituality, or beliefs in a higher power, may affect or be affected by pain. Some people find that religious observance or worship calms and soothes them, thereby decreasing perceptions of pain. For others, the social interaction offered by organized religious groups provides a strong support network and social outlet. Still others may feel abandoned and isolated if they believe that their faith has failed them.

Pain and Depression

Feeling some degree of frustration and discouragement is common when people are coping with cancer-related pain. Clinical depression, a treatable condition, occurs in about 25 percent of people with cancer and in about 80 percent of people with unrelenting chronic pain. It causes a person to feel hopeless, unmotivated, and less able to follow treatment demands. Some research also suggests that people with cancer who are also depressed recover more slowly from their illness.

About Depression

What to look for:
- persistent sad or "empty" mood almost every day for most of the day
- loss of interest or pleasure in ordinary activities
- eating problems (loss of appetite or overeating) or significant weight loss or gain
- sleep disturbances (insomnia, early waking, or oversleeping)
- noticeable restlessness or being "slowed down" almost every day
- decreased energy, or fatigue almost every day
- feelings of guilt, worthlessness, helplessness
- difficulty concentrating, remembering, making decisions
- thoughts of death or suicide, or attempts at suicide

Clinical depression may be diagnosed if a person has either of the first two symptoms along with at least one of the other symptoms during a two-week period.

What to do:
- Talk with your doctor or nurse about your depression and the possible ways to treat it.
- Seek help through counseling and support groups.
- Increase the amount of contact you have with other people.
- Schedule activities that are pleasant.
- Use prayer or other types of spiritual support.
- Use a problem-solving approach to tackle some of the day-to-day problems that are contributing to your feelings of depression.

Do not:
- Keep feelings inside—if pain is causing your depression, talk about it.
- Blame yourself for feelings of depression.

When to Notify Your Health Care Team about Depression
Contact your doctor or nurse if any of the following occur:
- you have thoughts of suicide
- you cannot eat or sleep and feel uninterested in activities of daily living for several days
- nothing you do seems to help, even those strategies that have worked in the past
- you persistently feel unable to enjoy anything

Depression can occur as a side effect of some medicines, or it can be caused by unrelieved pain. Depression can also develop as a response to the treatment and diagnosis of cancer. People in pain are more likely to become depressed than those who are not in pain.

Depression often affects sleep, appetite, and energy level. It may rob a person of the pleasure in life. It also tends to intensify a person's perception of pain; people with cancer who are clinically depressed report greater pain severity than those who are not depressed. Researchers note that patients who were depressed before a diagnosis of cancer report more intense pain than those who were not depressed before learning of their disease.

Depression should not be considered an acceptable or inevitable side effect of pain. It can be treated effectively with medication, counseling, or a combination of both. Antidepressant medications are prescribed by psychiatrists, primary care doctors, nurse practitioners, or oncologists. Effective treatment can help improve an individual's ability to cope with cancer and can even increase decision-making abilities.

The symptoms of clinical depression are listed on the previous page. Talk to your caregiver and health care team if your sad mood lasts more than two weeks or interferes with your ability to carry on day-to-day activities. If the help of a trained counselor or therapist is needed, your doctor or nurse will help you find a therapist who is trained to help people with chronic illnesses such as cancer.

Pain and Anxiety

Anxiety and fear are normal responses to unpleasant and stressful situations—such as being in pain—and are common feelings in people with cancer. Anxiety also may be caused by changes in family roles and responsibilities, loss of control over events in life, changes in body image, uncertainty about the future, and concerns about suffering, pain, and the unknown.

Some people may not always be able to identify their own feelings of anxiety. They may think they are just worried. Before they realize what

About Anxiety

What to look for:
- feelings of panic
- feeling as though you are losing control
- difficulty solving problems
- feeling excitable
- anger or irritation
- increased muscle tension
- trembling and shaking
- headaches, upset stomach, diarrhea, constipation
- sweaty palms, racing pulse, difficulty breathing

What to do:
- Talk with your doctor or nurse about your anxiety and possible ways to treat it.
- Talk about feelings and fears that you or family members may be having.
- If possible, identify the situations that may be adding to the anxiety.
- Solve day-to-day problems that are causing you stress.
- Engage in pleasant, distracting activities.
- Seek help through counseling and support groups.
- Use prayer or other types of spiritual support.
- Try deep breathing and relaxation exercises several times a day (see chapter 7).

Do not:
- Keep feelings inside—if pain is causing your anxiety, talk about it.
- Blame yourself for feelings of anxiety and fear.

When to Notify Your Health Care Team about Anxiety
Contact your doctor or nurse if:
- you have feelings of panic
- you are having trouble breathing, are sweating, and feel very restless
- you experience trembling, twitching, and feeling "shaky"
- your heart rate and pulse have rapidly increased
- you have problems sleeping several nights in a row

is happening, they may feel out of control. If you feel you are so anxious that you no longer cope well with day-to-day life, it may be a good idea to seek help outside the family. Ask your doctor or nurse about your symptoms of anxiety. An assessment can be made to determine whether the side effects of cancer or its treatments may be causing the anxiety. Changes in treatment, antianxiety medication, or counseling may help.

The Impact of Pain on Relationships

Support from Friends and Family

According to some research, people with cancer who tap into a solid network of friends and family tolerate pain better than those who confront their pain alone. In fact, this support may play a critical role in helping people with cancer cope with pain. In one study involving women with recurrent breast or gynecological cancer, researchers found a strong association between increased social activity and decreased pain levels. The study also noted that as pain increased, people's sense of confidence in how they were doing and their ability to socialize decreased. It's important to try to keep up some contact with others; if you have little social support, you may feel isolated and experience more pain.

Changing Relationships

Cancer and cancer pain can change relationships within and outside the family. Friends and family who are worried or uncomfortable may keep their distance when you most need their support. Friends may not keep in touch for a variety of reasons. Some people are afraid of cancer or pain and often unknowingly withhold physical affection. Others just don't know what to say or how to act. Friends and family may withdraw from you if you are unable to participate in previously shared activities because they do not want to remind you of what you are unable to do right now.

However, increasing physical and social contact may help buffer your pain. Some people prefer to face their pain and illness alone, but most can benefit from the comfort and support of friends and family.

Being open with your friends and family—and encouraging your caregiver to share an appropriate level of information with them about

Helping People with Cancer Cope with Feelings about Pain

Caregivers might find it helpful to keep in mind the following tips for helping those with cancer cope with the complicated feelings they may be having about cancer and cancer pain:

- Help the person with cancer deal with the emotional impact of pain. Some people try to deal with pain by pretending that it doesn't exist. That denial can be harmful if it leads to situations where the illness is made worse, such as by avoiding treatment or participating in activities that are physically harmful.
- Support the efforts of the person with cancer to live as normal a life as possible.
- Create a climate that encourages communication. Talk about important or sensitive topics in a manner and place that are calm and conducive to open discussion—not in the midst of a crisis or an argument.
- Be available. One of the most important messages you can communicate is, "If you want to talk about this, I'm willing to listen and talk." However, leave the timing up to the person in pain. To the greatest extent possible, the person with cancer should make decisions on what feelings to share and when, how, and with whom to share them. By not pressing the issue, you allow the person to retain control over part of life at a time when many other things feel beyond his or her control.
- Understand that men and women often communicate differently, and make allowances for those differences. Women sometimes express their feelings more openly than men in our society. If you're a male caregiver and the person with cancer is a woman, be aware when she shares feelings. You may find yourself giving advice when she just wants someone to listen and be understanding.

    If you're a female caregiver and the person with cancer is male, be aware that he may express his feelings differently than you would. Pay special attention when he talks about things that are important to him. It may be helpful to openly discuss differences in how men and women express feelings and how the person wants to be supported.

your health, your needs, and any limitations—may help everyone understand how you're feeling and how they can remain involved in your life.

Caregivers' Important Roles
Family members and friends who assume caregiving responsibilities play important roles for many people with cancer pain. Your caregiver will often give you pain medicines and make sure health professionals are informed about and responsive to your pain. Caregivers may also provide

help with routine activities, such as cooking, cleaning, and shopping. In addition to helping in practical ways, caregivers can provide encouragement, offer emotional support, and share experiences and knowledge learned from major problems faced in their own lives. Caregivers may also offer their opinions about treatment-related decisions.

Caregivers can greatly influence your pain experience by offering both physical and emotional support. And a caregiver's outlook can have a significant impact on your attitude about pain relief. If caregivers believe that pain can be relieved, you are more likely to believe it too.

Caregivers feel many pressures. The responsibility of caring for a person in pain can be both mentally and physically exhausting, and may lead to sadness and feelings of helplessness and anger because they cannot do more. Caregivers may even feel guilty for being angry. If unrecognized or ignored, these feelings can compromise their ability to help.

You are also coping with the physical effects and psychological and social challenges of cancer and pain. Depending on others to care for you may make you feel guilty, angry, or depressed by a loss of independence. These emotions are normal, but they can cause strain between you and your caregivers.

Working together will help everyone. Openly discussing needs and concerns will make sure that everyone has realistic expectations. Let others know what you need and want. Both you and your caregivers should be clear about what you need and expect and how much help a caregiver can provide so there is no confusion about roles.

Asking for Help

Cancer is a complicated set of diseases that require the attention of a variety of specialists, including surgeons, medical oncologists, radiation oncologists, and teams of support staff. People with cancer may need the services of a mental health professional to help confront the psychological, emotional, and social implications of cancer and cancer pain.

Psychosocial support services are provided by clinicians who understand how cancer and cancer pain affects patients and families and how to help them confront difficult issues related to the illness. These professionals include family counselors, psychologists, therapists, social workers, nurses, and chaplains. Counseling is offered for individuals, couples, families, or in a group setting. A decision about counseling will likely be affected by a number of factors, such as what services are available and their cost. Ask your health care team about the resources available at your hospital. You can also contact the American Cancer Society (800-ACS-2345; http://www.cancer.org) to find out about sources of support available in your community. The *Resources* section of this book also contains contact information for groups and organizations that provide support.

When to Seek Counseling

Your own feelings may be the most useful guide for deciding whether to seek counseling. At the beginning of a cancer experience, most people go through a period of turmoil, which includes feelings of anxiety, sadness, and fear about the future. You may have questions about why this has happened to you and the meaning of your life. You may feel worried about your job, finances, insurance, and other practical matters. Gradually, as you get through the first stages of treatment, you will find ways to address your concerns.

Cancer-related pain may make your decisions and feelings more complicated. Close family members or friends can play a major part in helping you figure out how to deal with cancer pain. An objective observer, such as a counselor or therapist, can identify new and effective ways of coping with cancer and cancer pain.

Chronic feelings of hopelessness, anxiety, and fear will deprive you of the energy you need to cope. If you feel very sad or worried much of the time or are unable to make decisions, a counselor or other mental health professional can usually help. Talking with a professional may allow you to find quicker resolutions to problems or challenges than you would by struggling on your own. Your goal will be to gradually feel more in control of your situation and be able to focus on managing your health and your pain.

Finding Support

There are many resources available for people with cancer pain and their families. Support can come from family and friends as well as health care professionals, support groups, or a place of worship. Asking for support is one way you can take control.

You may live alone or feel lonely. If you do not have support from friends and family, you can find it elsewhere. There are others in your community who need your companionship as much as you need theirs. The mutual support of other people with cancer can be a powerful source of comfort. The *Resources* section of this book lists organizations and groups that offer support to people with cancer and/or pain and their families and caregivers.

Support Groups

People who join a patient support group can learn new coping skills and expand their social network. According to some studies, those who participate in group therapy may experience less psychological distress and pain.

The purpose of a support group is to help people share their concerns with others and to learn new ways of solving problems. Participants can expect to learn more about coping with cancer and get new ideas from others in the same situation—for example, how they have managed episodes of pain.

Support groups for people with cancer may meet in hospital settings, within a community agency, a family service agency, or even in a patient's home. They vary widely in size and format, as well as duration. Some groups are small and meet weekly without a scheduled agenda, while others meet monthly and offer information, teach coping skills, help reduce anxiety, and provide a place to share common concerns and emotional support.

Groups can be organized by professionals or by people who have had cancer. Professionals include oncology social workers or nurses, psychologists, psychiatrists, psychiatric nurses, marriage and family therapists, or clergy. Professionals should be licensed in their respective fields and have skills in group "facilitation."

Self-Help Groups

Self-help groups are typically run by nonprofessionals who have been affected by a particular situation, such as people with cancer who have had pain. People who relate to your experience firsthand often have treatment-related tips that will be helpful to you. They may offer a home remedy that is helpful with managing pain, for example. People with cancer may feel freer to express exactly how they feel in self-help groups that do not include family members. Family members can benefit from sharing their feelings, fears, and anxieties with other families affected by cancer.

Self-help groups also give those recovering or recovered from cancer an opportunity to aid others who have cancer. With some training, many people with cancer who become group leaders find that it helps them as well; they get an opportunity to become group counselors or facilitators.

Choosing when to participate in a support group is important. Some people are not ready to join a support group when they are diagnosed with cancer. It may be difficult to participate if you are in continuous pain. Hearing the stories of other people with cancer can be overwhelming and upsetting. If you try a group and it doesn't feel right, you may want to try again at another time or try a different group.

For those who cannot attend meetings or appointments, counseling over the telephone is offered by certain organizations (see the *Resources* at the back of this book for more information). Some people prefer the privacy of online support groups. (Keep in mind, however, that Internet chat rooms and message boards are not the best source of cancer information, especially if they are not monitored by trained professionals or experts.) Regardless of the group's structure, you should feel comfortable in the group and with the facilitator. If you have any fears or uncertainties before entering a group, discuss them with the group's facilitator.

Individual Therapy

Individual psychotherapy or counseling has also been shown to help patients reduce anxiety and depression, factors that can intensify pain (see chapter 1 for more information). During individual counseling, people meet one-to-one with a counselor or therapist. The counselor's first objective is to determine specific concerns that need to be addressed. He or she will also want to find out how you have dealt with problems in the past, including what is or is not working now. The counselor will help you make sure that your greatest needs are considered.

You may talk about different ways to approach a situation before acting on your first impulse. Don't become impatient or frustrated if a strategy doesn't seem to work at first. Problem-solving sometimes requires complex solutions, and progress may come gradually. Your personality, relationships among family members, ability to be flexible and try new things, feelings about your situation, and the effects of other life events all influence the counseling process and your ability to resolve challenges.

Here are just a few of the many different types of individual therapy:

- **Cognitive therapy** is directed at changing behavior by addressing the repetitive, negative thoughts that influence actions. With this type of therapy, people learn to reprogram harmful internal messages and create positive thoughts to change behavior.
- **Client-centered therapy** focuses on people's feelings and current experiences. The therapist in this setting encourages people to lead the sessions while providing empathy and support. The goal is to help people help themselves.
- **Psychodynamic therapy** is geared toward changing lifelong personality patterns by uncovering the connections between current emotional reactions and early childhood experiences. This is usually longer-term therapy that focuses on the underlying causes of a problem.

Family Therapy

Because cancer and cancer pain affect all family members, some health care professionals favor family counseling as an ideal way for families to address their anxieties and worries. People with cancer often state that lack of communication in their families is a problem. Changes in responsibilities can cause resentment and anxiety, and some family members may not feel comfortable openly discussing their feelings.

Family therapy focuses on relationship patterns, and all family members may be involved in therapy sessions. A counselor involved in this type of

Is Family Counseling Right for You?

One of the ways to decide whether to seek family counseling is to think about what is happening in your family. Could your family benefit from talking openly in a neutral setting about feelings and concerns? As you consider family counseling, you may want to ask yourself the following questions:

- Can I talk to my partner and loved ones about how I feel?
- Are my partner and loved ones able to listen to what I am saying, or does it seem to be too painful for them?
- Does it help to talk to my partner when things are going badly?
- Do we always end up in a fight about how we are reacting?
- Do my children seem worried?
- Do they tell me how they feel?
- Are my children misbehaving more than usual?
- Is it harder to get them to listen?
- Do my children seem sad or lonely?
- Do they seem unable to enjoy being together as a family?
- Are they fighting among themselves more often?
- Are their grades suffering?
- Am I getting more complaints from my child's school?
- Are my children going backwards in their development? (For example, are they having more difficulty separating from you, maintaining toilet training, being unable to play by themselves, or being unusually dependent on you?)
- Is my family able to accept help from others?
- Do I resent that people outside the immediate family seem happy?
- Do I feel angry a lot of the time that others don't have this burden to deal with?
- Are financial or insurance problems interfering with my ability to deal with my family?

therapy acts as a facilitator to help a family or couple communicate their feelings more effectively. Through family counseling, families learn to deal with changes within the family and discuss their feelings more comfortably.

For many people, change is difficult. Recognizing problems and understanding why you or family members behave in certain ways are important steps in learning how to talk openly and face potentially difficult realities when one member of the family has cancer and is experiencing cancer pain.

It is often easier for someone outside the family, such as a counselor, to help family members see a situation differently. Once that is accomplished, the family may be more able to support each other, rather than shutting each other out.

Choosing a Counselor

The two most important factors to consider when choosing a counselor or therapist are the person's experience in helping people who have cancer and cancer pain, and how comfortable you feel with that person. Professionals who work in cancer treatment centers tend to have more knowledge and experience with emotional responses to cancer than those who do not. Counselors with experience working with people with cancer have a framework for understanding your reactions and feelings and understand how to recognize normal responses and help you deal with your emotions.

Other important factors to consider in selecting a counselor are professional training and credentials. At a minimum, counselors should possess a master's degree in one of the counseling fields, along with appropriate certification or licensure. Counselors usually come from the fields of social work, psychology, psychiatry, psychiatric nursing, or pastoral counseling. But while credentials will demonstrate a person's formal education in a chosen field, they ideally should be backed up with experience working with people with cancer. Don't feel shy about asking about a counselor's experience and education. Professionals who are secure in their abilities know that people need the most knowledgeable source of help and should readily provide you with the information you request.

Some people with cancer believe that unless counselors have endured cancer, they will be of little help. While surviving cancer may add to the counselor's expertise, it is not essential. Counselors who have worked with people with cancer have gained valuable experience. We have all experienced crises and losses as a normal part of life.

Consider how you feel when you first meet with a counselor or therapist. Does it feel safe to share your concerns with this person? Do you trust the counselor's ability to help you? Do you feel that the counselor listens well and understands you as an individual? Do you think your

A variety of professionals offer counseling:

- **Social workers** help people with cancer and their families adjust to the practical and emotional problems related to illness. They focus on social functioning, which includes helping people with community and financial resources, health care systems, employment concerns, legal and ethical issues, insurance coverage, child care, and other needs. Oncology social workers specialize in helping people manage concerns related to cancer and work closely with health care professionals who treat people with cancer.

- **Psychologists** are licensed professionals who usually have doctoral degrees (PhD, PsyD, EdD) and provide counseling and psychotherapy, testing if needed, teaching, and consultation. They may also do research. Psycho-oncologists are psychologists who are experienced in counseling people with cancer and their loved ones. They can help people adjust to illness, manage anxiety and depression, and cope with other emotional problems.

- **Psychiatrists** specialize in the field of medicine that focuses on the diagnosis and treatment of mental illness. Psychiatrists are licensed doctors (MDs) who can prescribe medication to treat psychiatric illness and conduct psychotherapy.

- **Marriage and family therapists** are mental health professionals trained in couples counseling and family therapy. They are licensed in many states to work with people who have problems in their relationships, marriages, or families. They have graduate training (a master's or doctoral degree) in marriage and family therapy and at least two years of clinical experience. If your state does not offer licensure, ask if the therapist is certified in marriage and family therapy from the American Association of Marriage and Family Therapists (AAMFT).

- **Licensed professional counselors** provide mental health and substance abuse counseling in a variety of settings. They are licensed in many states to work with individuals, families, groups, and organizations. They have at least a master's degree and are trained in understanding human growth, development, and psychosocial problems.

- **Pastoral counselors** focus on spiritual beliefs to reach emotional healing and growth. Certified pastoral counselors have mental health and religious training.

- **Psychiatric/mental health nurses** conduct assessments of patients' psychosocial and physical needs; offer assistance with basic life skills; and provide individual, group, and family counseling, training, and education. They have a master's degree and are certified as nurses who specialize in mental health services.

You can get referrals by asking members of your health care team or by contacting professional organizations for names of psychotherapists who specialize in the area. Oncology units of hospitals sometimes have staff counselors.

family could relate easily to this person? Trust your instincts. If somehow you just don't feel comfortable after a few sessions, it's probably wise to try someone else. You will know when you have found the right match.

Why Do Some People Need Help and Others Don't?

One of the concerns for people needing support services is how they feel about asking for help. Some people have the idea that they should know how to handle every problem or challenge, even though they have never been confronted with a crisis like cancer. Sometimes people feel that needing help with a problem is a sign of weakness. Asking for help can be a sign of strength. Learning about what you might expect from yourself and other family members can help you solve problems more quickly and effectively than attempting to solve them alone.

Feel free to ask for early help in coping with cancer and cancer pain. During periods of active treatment, you may be in too much pain or feel too overwhelmed to seek help. If you are experiencing a great deal of pain, it may be harder for you to feel in charge of your situation. By enlisting help coping with cancer and pain early in the process, you can focus more energy on your treatment for cancer or pain.

For some people, the idea of getting professional help for emotional or family problems is not acceptable. They feel that somehow needing help means that they are "weak," unstable, or even "crazy." While everyone sometimes feels as though they should be able to manage just about anything, there will be times during your cancer experience that telling yourself to be strong just does not work.

Learning what you need to know about cancer medically along with what you can expect of yourself and your family socially and emotionally takes time. Sorting through the medical aspects of cancer is an enormous challenge in itself, and people with cancer may not have the energy to cope with the added burden of pain and accompanying emotional issues by themselves. They may ignore these issues until life feels more settled. This is understandable, since people can only cope with so much at one time.

How You Will Know if Counseling Is Working

You will know counseling is helping you and your family if you can answer yes to at least some of the following questions:

- Are you gaining more insight into your problems?
- Is it becoming easier to keep the situation in perspective?
- Do you feel like you have more options?
- Do you feel less anxious or worried?
- Has your concentration improved?
- Is it easier to make decisions?
- Do you have a clear idea of what needs work immediately and what can wait until later?
- Are you increasingly in control over how you are feeling and behaving?
- Has your performance improved at work or home?
- Can the counselor give you some idea of how long you will need help?
- Can you tell your doctor or nurse how counseling is helping?

Ask your family members the same questions if they are involved in counseling. If your answers to these questions seem positive, you are probably on the right track. If you don't feel good about your answers to these questions, discuss them with your counselor. It may be that you expect different things than your therapist does or that you misunderstand the counseling process in some way. It may also mean that you need to find someone who is a better match for your personality or situation.

Finding the right counselor or therapist may take time and effort, but counseling often offers great benefits for you and your family.

But struggling alone is unnecessary. Asking for help understanding and anticipating what is to come is best for you and your family. Give yourself the benefit of other people's experiences and insights so that you can approach your situation with as much hope and optimism as possible. That way you can manage your illness and get on with your life.

Realize that it may not be possible to control everything going on in your life. Having cancer or cancer-related pain is new territory and it will take some time to discover what strategies work best for you. Don't be hesitant or afraid to seek the support you need in order to feel better.

Will Insurance Pay for Counseling and Therapy Services?

Insurance benefits for counseling services depend on your particular health plan and its coverage for mental health services. Most health plans offer at least some coverage for counseling, but it is often limited. Some policies only pay for a few counseling or psychotherapy sessions or may limit your choices of which professionals you can visit.

If you don't understand your coverage, ask a hospital or clinic social worker for help. A social worker can usually help you find accurate information about your plan and what is covered. A hospital's billing department may also examine your policy and determine your coverage. Social workers often know about services in the community that adjust their fees according to your income. Some hospitals and community health centers even offer free counseling or support groups.

CHAPTER 3

Achieving Effective Pain Control

A new nurse was recently hired to work in a hospital oncology unit. She admitted that she had not worked in this area before, but was willing to take the challenge. When Mrs. Allen in room 231 asked for pain medicine while she was laughing on the phone, the new nurse expressed her disbelief that Mrs. Allen was asking for pain medicines. "She was laughing on the phone; she wasn't having pain," was her comment. Of course, the nurses who had worked with great effort to get Mrs. Allen's severe pain under control knew that she was having pain. Thus began the long road of teaching the new nurse about oncology and the needs of people with cancer.

PROVIDING KNOWLEDGE AND DISPELLING MISINFORMATION about pain and pain relief is so important that this section of the book is devoted to the topic. If so many barriers did not stand between pain and pain relief, many people with cancer would be able to reduce pain to levels that do not detract significantly from their lives.

Myths and Misconceptions about Cancer Pain

The following myths and misunderstandings among both health care professionals and people with cancer represent barriers and obstacles to effective pain treatment. Exploring and dispelling these myths is essential to achieving adequate pain control.

Myth 1: People Become Addicted to Pain Medications

Probably the most widespread misconception about cancer pain treatment is that pain medications will lead to addiction, or uncontrollable drug craving, drug-seeking, and drug use. This worry prevents many patients from taking medications prescribed to relieve pain. The fact is that people who take cancer pain medicines as prescribed by their health care team rarely become addicted to them.

If you have a history of substance abuse or other concerns about addiction, share them with those who are caring for you (see chapter 9 for important information for people with a history of substance abuse). These fears should not prevent you from using medicines to relieve your pain.

Even many medical professionals, including doctors, lack thorough knowledge about pain treatment and addiction and continue to work under the impression that the use of opioids (strong pain relievers) may lead to drug addiction. Medical training often focuses on treating diseases, not on relieving symptoms. If your doctor is reluctant to prescribe pain medication when necessary, you may want to seek another opinion.

Myth 2: Taking Too Much Pain Medication Will over Time Decrease Its Effectiveness

Another misconception is that your body will become "immune" to the effects of the pain medicine. This fear may cause you to hold off on taking opioids or to save the strongest opioids for when pain becomes more severe. Keep in mind that it is easier to prevent pain and keep it under control than relieve pain after it has become severe.

Some people who take opioids for pain may find that over time they need to take larger doses. This may be due to an increase in pain or the development of drug tolerance. Drug tolerance occurs when your body gets used to the medicine you are taking and your medicine does not relieve the pain as well as it once did. Many people do not develop a tolerance to opioids. Usually small increases in the dose or a change in the kind of medicine will help relieve the pain for those who have developed drug tolerance. Increasing the doses of opioids to relieve increasing pain or to overcome drug tolerance does *not* lead to addiction.

Myth 3: Pain Is a Normal Part of Having Cancer

While many people with cancer experience pain, pain should not be considered normal or an unavoidable consequence of having cancer. Pain is not a necessary part of cancer, and it takes a major physical and emotional toll on a person. Any pain should be addressed aggressively, quickly, and with all of the resources available to your health care team. Remember that in almost all circumstances, when pain does occur, it can be controlled.

Myth 4: Pain Means that the Cancer Is Growing

Pain is not necessarily a sign that cancer is progressing or is incurable. Pain is not an inevitable consequence of cancer, but it may occur at any time during the course of illness and for any number of reasons. Even people whose condition is stable and whose life expectancy is long may feel pain.

Many things can cause aches and pains besides the progression of cancer. Headaches or backaches can be caused by things other than cancer, for example. Some pain can be caused by side effects of the cancer treatment. For example, people who receive chemotherapy may have sores in their mouth that are very painful, and those who have radiation to the lower abdomen can have cramping with diarrhea or develop a painfully sore rectum. Sometimes people with cancer may have pain because of the location of a tumor, which will not always mean that the cancer has progressed.

Myth 5: Pain Can't Be Treated

Some people simply believe that pain is just something they have to "deal" with. They think pain is inevitable and that all they can do is accept their fate. There are very few cases of pain that cannot be reduced so that the person in pain can function and enjoy life. Cancer pain can almost always be reduced safely, effectively, and sometimes quickly using relatively simple methods.

Myth 6: Doctors Don't Understand Pain

It is your right as a patient to receive assistance in pain management, and your doctor should be able to help relieve your pain. Some doctors and other members of the cancer care team may not be adequately trained to assess and treat cancer-related pain, or they may not understand the urgency and importance of pain relief in the larger scheme of cancer treatment. If your doctor or nurse does not understand and care for your pain, it's important that you seek further help from someone else. Concerned and knowledgeable doctors and nurses can achieve good pain control for almost all of their patients. To do so, they must be aware of your situation and the factors involved in your pain. You are in the best position to provide them with the necessary information about your pain.

Myth 7: Good Patients Don't Complain

Some people think they are being a burden or difficult if they talk about being in pain. Sometimes people are afraid that their health care professionals will think they are exaggerating their pain or being cowardly. Although there are effective options for controlling pain, some people endure it needlessly rather than ask their health care teams to prescribe stronger or different medications or to try other treatments if the current drug therapy program is not working. People with cancer can actually help their doctors and nurses by explaining the details of their pain so the health care team can determine the best way to treat it.

Myth 8: Focusing on the Pain May Be a Distraction from Treating the Cancer

Some believe that by not "making waves" about pain, they will get more attention and better cancer treatment, fearing that doctors and nurses might focus on treating their pain over treating their cancer. Both pain and cancer can be treated at the same time. In fact, pain may make it very difficult for people to comply with cancer treatment—the very treatment that holds the promise for curing their disease and relieving their pain. Telling your health care team about pain will not compromise the quality of your cancer treatment (see chapter 4 for more information on describing your pain).

Myth 9: People Should Be Able to "Tough it Out"

Some people believe that they should be able to put up with pain. Factors such as their family or cultural background may have instilled the belief that acknowledging pain makes a person weak. However, tolerating pain can actually make a person weak, both physically and emotionally. Unrelieved pain causes a decrease in appetite, disturbed sleep, and diminished physical activity, and pain can quickly drain your energy. Pain should be treated as soon as possible.

Myth 10: Pain Medications Cause Unpleasant Side Effects

Some pain medications can cause side effects, but many of those side effects can be managed or prevented, or diminish with time. The potential for side effects is no reason to avoid using these highly effective pain relievers. Opioids almost always cause some degree of constipation, but drinking lots of water, eating a high-fiber diet, and using laxatives and stool softeners will counteract the constipating effects. Opioids also cause many people to become drowsy or to fall asleep (which might actually be related to the fact that pain has kept them from getting adequate rest). This effect usually diminishes within a few days after drug therapy begins.

Occasionally, patients become dizzy or feel confused when they take opioids. If this happens to you, tell your nurse or doctor. These side effects may disappear on their own or may be relieved by changing the dose or type of medication you take. Some people fear that opioids will make them "high" and make them lose control. These drugs can make you feel "spacey" and "out of it" for a short time, but your body will adjust to these changes.

Sometimes opioids cause nausea and vomiting at first. These side effects usually disappear after a few days or can be managed with anti-nausea drugs or by changing medications or doses. If you experience side effects from your pain medicine, notify your doctor or nurse immediately so they can take steps to bring you relief.

The Importance of Communication

To receive the most effective pain treatment, you must be willing to discuss your pain clearly, accurately, honestly, and on a regular basis with members of your health care team and with caregivers at home. Everyone experiences and deals with pain differently. Even the way people talk about the type or intensity of their pain and discomfort varies, so it is important for you to describe your unique experience of pain. Many people find that talking about pain in specific terms is difficult, but the more information you can give to your doctor or nurse, the more likely a solution will be found. Telling a doctor or family member that "it hurts" is only the beginning of the description of your pain.

Communicating with Your Health Care Team

The first and most critical step in communicating with your health care team is to make certain that your doctor, nurse, and other members of your health care team are aware of your pain and how it affects you. Because pain is such an individual experience, you are the best judge of your pain and the consequences it has in your life. Only you know how much pain you feel, what relieves it, what makes it worse, and how your pain-relief needs change over time.

When discussing your pain with your health care team, be as specific as possible (see chapter 4 for more information about describing and measuring your pain). Describe the pain's intensity, location, how long it lasts, how it changes, which pain-relief steps work and which do not, and the psychological effects the pain creates (for example, depression, anxiety, and worry). Armed with such information, the health care professional who is in charge of your pain treatment can design a plan to meet your needs. Together, you can map out the steps you will take toward relief, including medications, nondrug therapies, or special procedures.

Sometimes finding the right pain solution takes several attempts, regardless of a health care team's skill and knowledge. The process may require time and may be frustrating for patients, family, and health professionals. But in the long run, continuing to discuss your pain-relief needs with your health care team is likely to improve your pain relief and your quality of life.

Many concerned and compassionate health care providers are trained to focus on cancer treatment, but some simply do not realize that relieving pain is a crucial part of cancer treatment. Few medical schools include education about the importance of treating chronic pain that often accompanies cancer and the best methods for doing so. Patients and their caregivers must make sure their doctors and nurses view pain seriously and take all necessary steps to relieve it.

Cancer care is typically provided through a team approach, in which the skills and talents of various medical professionals are applied to different aspects of treatment. But do not assume that everyone on your health care team knows about your case or your pain-control needs. Consider speaking with each team member about your pain and pain-management needs so that you understand how each may be able to help you. When all members of the team communicate well and work together, efforts at pain relief are more likely to succeed. Together, you and your health care team can develop an effective plan for pain relief. Members of your health care team need to hear about what works to relieve your pain and what doesn't. Discussions about pain will not distract your health care team from treating the cancer, but will result in a better understanding of how the cancer and its treatment affect your body, potentially improving the treatment of your disease and symptom management. The best time to tell your doctor or nurse about pain is immediately after it begins, because pain is easier to treat when it first occurs than after it becomes troublesome or severe.

Communicating with Caregivers

Communicating with caregivers is essential to your care. Caregivers may play an important part in your pain-management program (see chapter 2 for more information) by offering encouragement and emotional support, helping you describe your pain to health care providers, making sure that you follow your pain treatment plan, and reporting changes in your behavior or attitude to a doctor or nurse. A caregiver can also become your advocate and act as a link between you and your health care providers, and may even become an active participant in the decision-making process. While you might want to be as independent as possible, there will be times when the help of others can be important.

Barriers to Communication

Many communication barriers can prevent patients from receiving adequate pain care. These may include language and cultural differences between patients and health care professionals (see chapter 9 for more information about cancer pain in culturally diverse groups), patients' inability or reluctance to discuss pain, and lack of recognition by health care workers about the importance of pain control.

Language Barriers

Because pain is best reported by the person who experiences it, the ability to communicate verbally with doctors, nurses, and other health care professionals is essential to ensuring that patients receive the best pain relief possible. Patients who speak a foreign language and have limited command of the English language may find it difficult to communicate with health care professionals who speak only English. They will not be able to describe their pain adequately and may not receive the appropriate amount of attention. If doctors and nurses do not understand their patients, they will not be able to assess pain accurately and therefore may not be able to formulate the most effective pain-management strategy.

People in pain may revert to their primary language when under stress. When there is a difference in language, the medical staff may have to rely on simple visual tools to assess a patient's pain and to gauge the effects of treatment. For example, health professionals may, with the help of a translator, help a patient devise a simple, two-language verbal rating scale that both can understand and use to measure pain and pain relief.

Hospitals typically have staff members who act as translators for patients who speak languages other than that of their health care team. Caregivers who understand both the language used by the health care team and the primary language of the patient may also serve as translators. In addition, patients who do not understand the language spoken by their health care team well should find out if printed instructions about cancer pain and pain control are available in their language.

Cultural Background

Cultural background—ethnicity, religious beliefs, personal values, morals, or family dynamics—can greatly influence how people cope with and talk about their pain. Culture influences not only how people perceive pain, but also how and even if they are willing to discuss it with health professionals and caregivers. Communication styles and general attitudes about both traditional and nontraditional forms of medical care are influenced by culture. Culture also has a major impact on how individuals view pain-relief measures (such as drug therapy) and how much pain they will endure before asking for help.

Pain Is Subjective

Each person perceives and deals with pain in a unique way. A level of pain that causes one person to cry out may cause another to become very quiet. People may describe their pain experiences quite differently. One might use the words "occasional" and "bearable," while another may describe a similar level of pain as "frequent" and "severe." People with cancer tend to underreport their own pain levels when meeting with doctors, often because they are more concerned about whether their cancer therapy is working than being pain-free. No objective test exists to measure how much pain a person has. Health care providers and caregivers must simply accept that patients are in as much pain as they say they are, which makes accurate assessment challenging. But while pain assessment is challenging, determining how much pain a person is in is important; it provides the health care team with a baseline from which to develop a treatment plan.

A pain-management plan cannot be effective if you fail to report pain. You have a right to the best pain control you can get. Decreasing your pain will allow you to continue to do the everyday things that are important to you.

- Speak out if someone offends you. When people are being insensitive, let them know.
- Explain your thoughts and fears to an understanding person, whether a friend or therapist. Talking to understanding people will show you that others empathize with you and can help you think through the impact of your emotions.
- Express your emotions as you wish. You may not want to share your emotions and feelings with everyone. It's okay to spend time alone, but be aware that there are people with whom you can talk.
- Sharing doesn't always mean talking. You may feel more comfortable writing about your feelings.
- Having a sense of control over what happens to you makes a difficult experience easier to manage. Gathering information about your pain, participating in treatment decisions, and knowing what to expect can counteract feelings that your situation is hopeless. It is not necessary to learn every detail, ask every question, and make all the decisions. You can gain control by making sure you have a health care team that you trust to recommend and provide the best care you need.
- Pain is in *your* body and is affecting *your* life. Therefore, it's up to you to determine your priorities and needs. Trust the members of your health care team and listen carefully to what they say. But before you decide on a pain-relief program, make sure you're informed enough to feel confident that the plan you and your health care team have structured is what's best for you. Explore and clarify every aspect of treatment before beginning.

Limited Knowledge and Time

Poor communication may occur if health care providers are inadequately trained to assess pain or are not familiar with the most current pain-management strategies. Some medical professionals may inaccurately judge a person's severity of pain and may not understand that a person in pain is less likely to comply with important cancer treatment instructions.

Many doctors are under great pressure to keep visits short and focus on cancer treatment and may therefore pay inadequate attention to a patient's pain. Some medical professionals simply may not realize the tremendous impact pain has on a person's life.

It's essential that you and your caregiver are clear about your pain and insist upon pain management if necessary.

When to Seek Additional Help

You should expect your health care team to take all necessary steps to relieve your pain and make you as comfortable as possible. But when prescribed pain-relief strategies do not succeed, talk frankly with your health care team members and make it clear that you require better pain relief and that you need more attention paid to your pain.

Feel free to ask to be referred to a pain specialist or a pain clinic. New developments in pain management occur regularly, and your health care team may simply not be familiar with all of them. A doctor who has your best interest at heart and has genuinely tried to help relieve your pain in a sensitive and caring manner should not hesitate to help you find other sources of pain control. If you are in pain and your doctor doesn't seem to take your situation seriously or does not offer alternatives, seek treatment elsewhere.

Pain programs or specialists can be located through a cancer center, a hospice, or the oncology department at a local hospital or medical center. The American Cancer Society and other organizations may also be able to provide information on pain specialists, pain clinics, or programs in your area. (See the *Resources* section of this book for more information.) It is your right to seek appropriate care to relieve pain, and ultimately it is up to you to ensure that you get the care you need and deserve.

CHAPTER 4

Describing and Measuring Your Pain

Howard first noticed the pain in his ribs on his left side when reaching for a plate in the cupboard. He didn't know what to make of it. He had been receiving hormone treatment for prostate cancer for over four years and because the new pain was so vague, he didn't know if it could be related. He wasn't scheduled to see his doctor for another month, and he was unsure if he could describe what the pain felt like if his doctor asked.

IN MOST CASES, YOU ARE THE BEST SOURCE OF INFORMATION about your pain, since only you can convey complete information about how bad the pain is, where it is located, which pain-control methods work, and which do not. No one else can guess about your pain experience.

Studies have found that doctors and nurses rarely rate pain at the same level of severity as patients do, more often rating patients' pain as less intense than the patients do. These findings highlight the importance of communication. Your health care team will have no way of knowing or understanding your pain unless you tell them. Because there is no reliable method to objectively measure pain, your health care team and caregivers at home will depend on you to keep them informed about your situation.

The "Language" of Pain

When talking with members of your health care team or with caregivers, it can be very helpful to use words and descriptions that clearly and specifically describe your pain. By communicating with your health care team in a "common language," you can provide reliable and consistent descriptions. This helps them make an accurate diagnosis of the causes of pain and decide which treatment options to prescribe.

In order for you—and others—to get a better understanding of your pain, ask yourself the following questions:

- **When did my pain begin?** It is important for your health care team to know about the onset of pain (when the pain first began). They can use this information to determine the source of pain and whether or not it is related to cancer. Pain that began before the diagnosis of cancer may be caused by factors other than cancer and may require a different type of treatment. The onset of pain may, on the other hand, be the reason you sought medical advice in the first place and what led to a diagnosis of cancer.

- **How long does my pain last?** Recall that acute pain appears suddenly (and often with great intensity) and disappears or diminishes quickly as well. Acute pain may be accompanied by a rapid heartbeat and an increase in blood pressure. If you experience acute pain, you may wince, grimace, or rub the affected area. In contrast, chronic pain is usually less intense but may have a longer duration—that is, it can last for a long time, in some cases many months (see chapter 1 for more information about acute and chronic pain).

- **Where (in what part of my body) do I feel pain?** Sometimes pain begins and remains in a single area. At other times it can radiate from one point to other parts of the body. The location of pain can change, and sometimes pain in one part of the body indicates that a problem exists elsewhere. For example, gallbladder disease is known to produce pain in the right shoulder. This is known as "referral" pain. The knowledge that pain may arise at sites other than the origin of the problem helps clinicians determine the cause and the type of treatment needed.

Words for Describing Pain

Flickering	Brief	Cruel	Exhausting	Hurting
Quivering	Momentary	Vicious	Wretched	Aching
Pulsing	Transient	Killing	Blinding	Heavy
Beating	Rhythmic	Tight	Cool	Sickening
Pounding	Periodic	Numb	Cold	Suffocating
Throbbing	Intermittent	Drawing	Freezing	Annoying
Pinching	Jumping	Squeezing	Continuous	Troublesome
Pressing	Flashing	Tearing	Steady	Miserable
Gnawing	Shooting	Pricking	Constant	Intense
Cramping	Tugging	Boring	Sharp	Unbearable
Crushing	Pulling	Drilling	Cutting	Nagging
Fearful	Wrenching	Stabbing	Lacerating	Nauseating
Frightful	Tender	Lancinating	Tingling	Agonizing
Terrifying	Taut	Hot	Itchy	Dreadful
Spreading	Rasping	Burning	Smarting	Torturing
Radiating	Splitting	Scalding	Stinging	
Penetrating	Punishing	Searing	Dull	
Piercing	Grueling	Tiring	Sore	

- **What does the pain feel like?** The quality of pain (what pain feels like) is described by words such as stabbing, burning, crushing, and many other terms. The quality of your pain is yet another factor that provides clues about the source of pain and what measures will be most effective in treating it. The *Words for Describing Pain* table above contains a wide selection of terms that can apply to pain. This list may help you to better describe your pain.
- **Is my pain constant, or does it change?** Your doctor or nurse will want to know about the pattern of pain, such as how often it comes and goes and whether its intensity, location, or duration changes during the day. They may also want to know whether routine actions such as moving your arms, breathing, swallowing, standing, sitting, or lying down trigger or ease your pain.

- **How severe is my pain?** Severity, or intensity, is often the most easily described component of pain. Your doctor or nurse may ask you not only to describe the severity of your pain in words (such as mild, moderate, or severe) but also to rate it on a special pain rating scale. For many people, using scales to describe the severity of pain is easier than using words to communicate about pain. (See the *Tools for Rating Your Pain* section on pages 67–69 of this book.)

Talking about Your Pain

As days went by, Howard's pain became more of a bother to him. His wife of thirty-five years, noticing him grimace while bending over, asked if everything was okay. He told her about the pain in his ribs and how frightened he was that it could be the cancer returning. She decided to accompany him to his doctor's visit.

Just talking about pain can be difficult. For many individuals, knowing how to describe the pain does not make it easier to talk about it, especially with people such as medical professionals. Some people in pain don't want to be a bother or don't want to disappoint the doctor. Some feel they are tough enough to live with the pain, while others don't want to admit they have pain for fear that it might mean their cancer has gotten worse or has spread. While some people can talk openly about their pain with a doctor or nurse, others find it easier to begin talking about it by confiding in someone they feel closer to.

Talking with Family Members and Caregivers about Pain

Family members and others who care for you are the second-best source of information about your pain and the effectiveness of pain treatment. Because caregivers spend more time with you than your health care team does, they are in a unique position to observe whether pain treatments appear to be effective and whether they cause side effects. They are most likely to notice any changes in your daily habits or ability to maintain routines, such as eating, sleeping, and moving.

Family members, friends, and caregivers can support you and better care for you if they understand your experience of pain, what measures relieve your pain, and what factors seem to make it worse. By understanding your experiences, they will know which changes to watch for and when to contact your health care team. They can also become important partners by reminding you to take your pain medications on time and by helping you evaluate and describe your pain.

Talking with Your Health Care Team about Pain

At the doctor's office, Howard's wife went with him into the exam room. "How have you been feeling?" asked the doctor. "Okay, I guess," was his response. "That's not exactly true," said his wife, who proceeded to explain his new pain to the doctor. Based on this information, his doctor ordered several tests. A small growth was discovered on one of his ribs. After discussion with his doctor, Howard and his wife decided he would undergo radiation treatment to the rib to relieve the pain.

The information you share with your health care team about your pain provides them with important clues about the source of pain and the best way to provide relief. In addition to sharing information about the key factors described earlier, let them know what pain treatments have typically worked best for you in the past, as well as how pain affects your mood and your level of psychological distress.

When you meet with doctors and nurses, let them know your goals and what you would like to happen as a result of your visit. Sometimes complete freedom from pain is a reasonable goal, while at other times getting enough relief to allow you to walk outside or to sleep comfortably at night may be more realistic. Explaining what you need helps your health care team make the best choices regarding your care. Make sure that you convey as much information as possible about your pain, even if some of it seems trivial. Let your health care team decide which details are important and which are not.

Pain should be assessed by your doctor or nurse at every office visit. Information about your pain will provide important clues about your treatment and if it is necessary to change your pain-control plans. (See *How Pain Is Measured* on page 61 for more information about pain assessments.) If your pain is causing problems for you, raise the issue when you meet with your doctor or nurse. Make sure that your health care team "hears" you.

Don't be afraid to take control of your treatment. During attempts to bring pain under control, you may become frustrated, anxious, or impatient. Express these sentiments to your health care team without fear that they may become angry or upset with you.

If you don't understand something, ask the doctor or nurse to repeat it or explain it more clearly. Good communication between patients and health care providers is known to improve the quality of care, and pain-relief efforts are more likely to succeed when you regularly describe your pain to your health care team. Remember that no question is stupid or silly when the subject is your health and well-being.

Many people find it helpful to take notes or to have a companion take notes for them when meeting with their health care team so they can fully concentrate on the information being discussed and so they won't forget any important information once they return home. Before seeking advice in person or over the telephone, list in advance the subjects you want to discuss. You may simply have a question about medication dose or timing, or you may be reporting the onset of new pain. In either case, you can help yourself by being prepared, knowing specifically what information you seek, and by being ready to supply the health care team with important information about your pain, the medications you take as well as how often, and how much

Questions to Ask Your Health Care Team about Pain

You might want to pose these questions to your health care team so you understand your pain and how to prevent and cope with it:

- What kind of pain am I likely to experience during or after cancer treatment?
- How do I know whether my pain is "normal" or a sign of some other complication?
- What kind of pain should I watch out for and report?
- Do I need pain medication?
- What kind of pain medication will alleviate my pain? What are the potential side effects?
- What if the pain medication isn't working? Should I take more?
- Can I become dependent on pain medication?
- How long will I have to take pain medication?
- What options do I have for pain control without medication?
- What else can I do to reduce pain?

relief you currently get from treatment. By supplying this information, you are more likely to avoid delays in treatment.

How Pain Is Measured

Pain assessment is an ongoing process during which a member of your health care team (usually a doctor or nurse) evaluates your pain and the effectiveness of pain-control measures. According to the guidelines of the Joint Commission on the Accreditation of Healthcare Organizations, hospitals are now required to monitor and document pain levels for all patients (see *Appendix B* for more information). Patients are asked to rate their pain at all stages of treatment using a numerical scale so pain can be tracked and attended to regularly.

The pain assessment process includes three components: an initial pain assessment; frequent reassessments as long as pain persists; and routine assessments for the occurrence of new pain. The overall goals of pain assessment are to create a detailed picture of how pain influences different aspects of your life, to identify the cause or causes of your pain, and ultimately to develop an effective pain-relief program to match your specific needs.

The Initial Pain Assessment

In addition to the radiation treatments, Howard was referred to a nurse specializing in pain management for evaluation. He and his wife prepared a list of questions prior to the appointment. They discussed how he had reacted to pain in the past and how pain medications might help him in the future if necessary. He was asked to describe his pain in his own words and to indicate the present level of his pain on a numeric scale so that the specialist could get an idea of the distress he was in. After hearing him describe his pain as a "3" on a scale from 0 to 10, the specialist decided to first try treatment with nonopioid pain relievers. Howard was instructed to call the office if the pain did not subside within three days.

Your Medical History

The initial pain assessment will most likely include creating or reviewing a comprehensive medical history that covers information such as your marital and job status, physical activity levels, recreational activities, support networks, social activities, strengths and weaknesses, and spiritual beliefs. The more information members of your health care team have about you as a whole person, the better able they will be to recommend treatments that might work best for you. You may also be asked if you have a reliable friend or family member who can take you to and from medical appointments and provide care at home, if necessary.

Your doctor or nurse will review your cancer history and the current status of your illness and treatment so that they can determine if all or part of your pain is the result of cancer or if it stems from other causes. Not all of the pain you feel is necessarily caused by cancer; it could come from other sources, such as injury, bruising, and conditions related to aging, such as arthritis.

Questions about Your Pain

As discussed earlier, your doctor or nurse will also ask questions about your pain, such as the onset, intensity, severity, quality, location, and the effects the pain has on your physical and emotional well-being. If you have been taking pain medications, the assessment will include an evaluation of their effectiveness. You will also be asked to report all other types of prescription and non-prescription medications you are taking, including herbal supplements or any other complementary or alternative methods you are using. (Complementary methods may be used along with standard therapy, but they are not given to cure disease. Alternative methods are promoted as cancer cures. They are unproven because they have not been scientifically tested, or were tested and found to be ineffective. See chapter 7 for more information about complementary methods that may help control pain.)

Physical Examination

The initial pain assessment may also include a thorough physical examination to identify any areas of tenderness and to monitor vital signs such as heart rate and blood pressure that may be affected during periods of pain.

Blood tests and other diagnostic procedures, such as x-rays, computerized tomography (CT) scans, and magnetic resonance imaging (MRI), may be ordered. While these tests don't reveal much information about the pain itself, they may indicate changes in bones and soft tissues that can help your health care team identify sources of pain and whether or not cancer cells have spread to other parts of the body. Such information helps health care providers decide on the best course of action to relieve your pain.

Psychological Assessment

Your doctor or nurse may perform a psychological assessment (also known as a psychosocial assessment) to determine how the pain affects your attitudes, moods, and emotions, and what impact it has on your daily activities. Physical pain often causes emotional changes such as anger, anxiety, fear, moodiness, inability to concentrate, and depression. You may be asked about your cognitive style—which describes how you view and interpret the world—and if you experienced any emotional disturbances before your diagnosis, such as depression, anxiety, or moodiness, or if you are generally overly concerned about health matters. You'll be asked how you typically cope with stress and pain, your expectations about pain management, the meaning of your pain to you and your family, significant past instances of pain and their effects on you, and your concerns about using controlled substances to manage pain. You will also be asked to report any previous or current drug or alcohol usage, which can affect the way a person reacts to pain-relief medications.

From the detailed information that you provide during the initial pain assessment, your health care team can develop a pain-relief program tailored specifically to your needs.

Preparing for a Pain Assessment

You can take a number of steps to ensure that you get the most from your pain assessment. One strategy is to review the variety of words for describing pain (see page 57) and select those that best describe your condition. It will also be helpful to write down a complete list of *all* of

continued on page 66

Suggested Preparation for a Pain Assessment

The following are tools you can use to get the most from a pain assessment and leave the meeting with all of the information you need to understand the various components of your pain-relief program.

Before the assessment:
- Write down any questions you'd like to ask.
- Write down specific goals you expect to reach at the pain assessment. (What do you want to happen as a result of your visit?)
- List any specific pain-related problems you're having, such as limited physical movement or emotional distress.
- Rate the intensity of your pain before and after you take pain medicine.
- Record the times when your pain was worst during several days before your visit.
- List any side effects caused by your medicine or by the pain itself.
- Record any measures, other than medication, you've tried to relieve pain and how well they worked (e.g., complementary pain treatments like hypnosis, relaxation, massage, or acupuncture).
- Make a list of all medications you currently take; include the dosage and the time(s) you take them. (As an alternative, you may want to bring all of your pill bottles with you.) For all pain medicines you are taking, list:
    1) the name of the medicine (either the trade name, which is capitalized, or the generic name)
    2) the amount of medicine in each pill (usually listed on the bottle in milligrams, or mg)
    3) how many pills you take for each dose
    4) how often you take medication
    5) how much medication you've taken in the past two days
    6) how long it takes the medicine to work
    7) the level of relief the medicine provides
    8) how long the relief lasts
    9) if the pain returns before the next dose, and if so how mild or severe it is
- Ask a companion to accompany you to the pain assessment to lend support and to help you record and interpret important information.
- Consider tape-recording the pain assessment. (Ask for permission ahead of time.)
- Bring a pad of paper and a pencil to write down important information.

During the assessment:
- Ask for an explanation of any word or phrase you don't understand. Your doctor or nurse should be able to explain medical terms in common language.
- If you don't understand something, ask the doctor or nurse to repeat it. Don't leave the doctor's office until you understand the reasons for all treatment decisions and expected outcomes.
- Don't be afraid to ask questions, no matter how trivial you think they are. Your questions are valid and important. Make sure all of your questions are answered.
- Communicate to your health care team about how much and what type of information you want them to give you.
- Tell the doctor or nurse the most effective way for you to receive information, such as through verbal explanations, written materials, or pictures. For some people, a combination of methods may work best when learning about complex medical subjects.
- Describe how pain interferes with your daily activities.
- Describe how you feel about the pain (e.g., angry, resigned, sad).
- Have your companion take careful notes, or take notes yourself if you are alone.
- Insist on privacy.

Questions to expect at a pain assessment:
- When did your pain begin?
- What does it feel like? Sharp, dull, throbbing? (See page 57 for words you might use to describe pain.)
- Where do you feel your pain?
- Does the location of your pain remain constant or does it move around?
- Is your pain constant? If not, how many times a day (or week) does it occur?
- How long does each period of pain last?
- How severe is your pain?
- Does your pain prevent you from doing your daily activities? Which ones?
- What makes your pain better or worse?
- What have you tried for pain relief and what were the results?
- What have you done in the past to relieve other kinds of pain?
- What medications for pain are you now taking?
- Does your current medication work, and how long does it last?
- Do you notice any side effects from your pain medication?

the medications you take, including the doses, times when you take them, and your opinion about how effective each one is. This list should include any dietary supplements, herbal remedies, and non-prescription medicines that you take. Many doctors recommend packing all of your pill bottles in a bag and taking them with you to the pain assessment.

Consider bringing a friend or close relative to the pain assessment. Ideally, your companion should be the person who is responsible for your overall care at home and who can serve as an advocate for you and provide aid when you are faced with important decisions. Your companion can also help you prepare questions before the assessment and take notes during the visit so you can focus completely on the information provided by your doctor or nurse. After the visit, a friend can help you review the results of the assessment and make sure that you adhere closely to the plan prepared by your health care team. If you prefer to attend a pain assessment alone, you may want to take careful notes or bring a tape recorder.

Some doctors or nurses may encourage you to bring family members to the initial pain assessment so they can understand the treatment plan, the importance of controlling pain, and how pain affects your life. They can also learn how to discuss pain with you, be more aware of pain-relief needs at home, and understand the effects of various pain medications, how to help you cope with side effects or problems, and when it is necessary to contact a doctor.

When the Person with Cancer Is Unable to Discuss Pain

Some people with cancer may be unable to discuss their pain or provide adequate information about their pain to doctors or nurses. For example, patients with hearing or vision difficulties, mental impairments, or decreased alertness due to opioids or pain itself may have difficulty remembering or communicating about when pain begins, how long it lasts, and what affects it. Some patients may be able to describe their pain by relying on simplified pain scales, such as a faces scale (see page 68). When a patient is unable to communicate, doctors are likely to rely more heavily on caregivers to observe and report behavioral changes that indicate decreased, constant, or increased pain. See chapter 9 for more information about pain assessment in children and in the elderly.

Tools for Rating Your Pain

Pain has many dimensions, all of which provide clues about its source and how it can be treated most effectively. There are a number of tools available to help you rate and describe your pain.

All of these types of scales can be useful in helping to answer questions such as:

- How bad is your pain when it is at its most intense?
- How bad is your pain most of the time?
- How bad is your pain when you feel it the least?

Numeric Scales

One of the most common types of pain rating tools is called a numeric scale. Numeric scales rely on numbers to help patients describe the intensity of their pain. Scales may range from 0 to 5, 0 to 10, or even 0 to 100, where 0 represents no pain and the highest number represents excruciating pain. Numeric scales can be used verbally or in a visual format (on a sheet of paper). Numbers are often displayed graphically along a line that is divided into segments. Patients can describe their pain level by marking a point along the line or by naming a number that best describes the severity of their pain, for example, "My pain is a 4 on a scale of 0 to 10." Numeric scales are often used to measure pain levels before and after a patient takes pain medication. They are easy to understand and generally provide an accurate measure of pain.

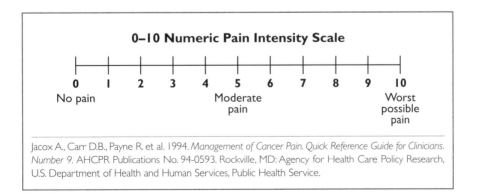

0–10 Numeric Pain Intensity Scale

0 — No pain   1   2   3   4   5 — Moderate pain   6   7   8   9   10 — Worst possible pain

Jacox A., Carr D.B., Payne R. et al. 1994. *Management of Cancer Pain. Quick Reference Guide for Clinicians. Number 9.* AHCPR Publications No. 94-0593. Rockville, MD: Agency for Health Care Policy Research, U.S. Department of Health and Human Services, Public Health Service.

Word Scales

Word scales present a patient with a continuum of words to choose from, such as "mild," "moderate," or "severe," or phrases such as "no pain," "a little pain," or "too much pain." For some patients, word scales are more effective than numeric scales for rating levels of distress. Word scales have been found to be particularly useful with elderly patients.

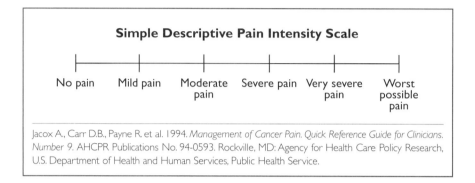

Simple Descriptive Pain Intensity Scale

No pain   Mild pain   Moderate pain   Severe pain   Very severe pain   Worst possible pain

Jacox A., Carr D.B., Payne R. et al. 1994. *Management of Cancer Pain. Quick Reference Guide for Clinicians. Number 9.* AHCPR Publications No. 94-0593. Rockville, MD: Agency for Health Care Policy Research, U.S. Department of Health and Human Services, Public Health Service.

The Faces Scale

Another way to rate pain nonverbally is with the faces scale, which consists of a series of faces that are smiling or frowning to various degrees or which show a neutral expression. To use the faces scale, patients point to the expression that most closely reflects their experience of pain. The faces scale is often used for children who are in pain but who cannot verbalize their sensations. It is also a useful tool for adults.

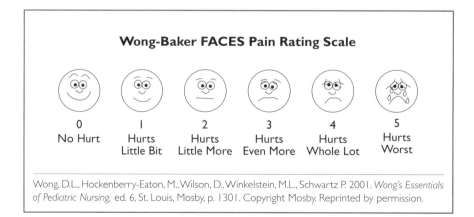

Wong-Baker FACES Pain Rating Scale

| 0 No Hurt | 1 Hurts Little Bit | 2 Hurts Little More | 3 Hurts Even More | 4 Hurts Whole Lot | 5 Hurts Worst |

Wong, D.L., Hockenberry-Eaton, M., Wilson, D., Winkelstein, M.L., Schwartz P. 2001. *Wong's Essentials of Pediatric Nursing*, ed. 6, St. Louis, Mosby. p. 1301. Copyright Mosby. Reprinted by permission.

Color Scales

Another way to communicate pain level is to select a color from a chart that best reflects the intensity of pain. Scales often begin with white (representing no pain) and end with red (representing severe or excruciating pain). Intermediate colors represent the range of pain levels in between.

The Brief Pain Inventory

The Brief Pain Inventory consists of questions designed to assess a patient's physical condition and psychological state, which can have a powerful effect on pain. This written form, which takes about fifteen minutes to complete, provides information about pain history, intensity, location, and quality. (See the following page.)

What to Do after the Initial Pain Assessment

Following the radiation treatment and daily doses of rofecoxib (Vioxx, a long-acting, aspirin-like medication), Howard's pain was diminished but still bothersome. He had difficulty getting out of bed without discomfort and was unable to pick up his young grandchildren without experiencing sharp pangs in his ribs. His wife phoned his doctor's office and scheduled a return visit. His doctor placed him on a stronger analgesic. Within a week his pain was almost gone.

Once a pain assessment has been completed, pain-relief measures should begin immediately if possible. A careful diagnostic workup should be completed even if some procedures cause pain since the results will determine the course of action that will relieve discomfort.

Your Pain Treatment Plan

Your doctor may recommend a variety of medications and other methods to treat your pain, including non-medical treatments (see chapter 7). Pain-relief medications are often prescribed in combinations to enhance

Brief Pain Inventory (Short Form)

Date: _____/_____/_____   Time:_____
Name: _____ _____ _____
                      Last   First   Middle Initial

1. **Throughout our lives, most of us have had pain from time to time (such as minor headaches, sprains, and toothaches). Have you had pain other than these everyday kinds of pain today?**

          1.   Yes   2.   No

2. **On the diagram, shade in the areas where you feel pain. Put an X on the area that hurts the most.**

Right   Left   Left   Right

3. **Please rate your pain by circling the one number that best describes your pain at its _worst_ in the last 24 hours.**

   0   1   2   3   4   5   6   7   8   9   10
   No   Pain as bad as
   pain   you can imagine

4. **Please rate your pain by circling the one number that best describes your pain at its _least_ in the last 24 hours.**

   0   1   2   3   4   5   6   7   8   9   10
   No   Pain as bad as
   pain   you can imagine

5. **Please rate your pain by circling the one number that best describes your pain on the _average_.**

   0   1   2   3   4   5   6   7   8   9   10
   No   Pain as bad as
   pain   you can imagine

6. **Please rate your pain by circling the one number that tells how much pain you have _right now_.**

   0   1   2   3   4   5   6   7   8   9   10
   No   Pain as bad as
   pain   you can imagine

their effectiveness. Be sure that your health care team knows about all of the medications you take and whether you can continue to use them after beginning therapy for pain. (See chapter 5 for more information about pain medicines and important warnings about alcohol, other medications, and side effects.)

Follow-up pain assessments should be conducted on a regular basis and should be scheduled every time you experience a new type of pain, or if an existing pain grows worse or changes noticeably in character. During follow-up pain assessments, your health care team will evaluate the effectiveness of pain-relief measures that were initiated after previous pain assessments. Based on the information you provide, your doctor will determine if changes in your pain are related to cancer, cancer treatment, or other factors, and will then decide if any changes (such as trying a new pain medication or increasing the dose of a current medication) should be made to your pain-management plan.

Communicating about Pain and Pain Relief

After beginning treatment for pain, it is important to stay in close touch with your health care team to report the results—or lack of results—of your treatment. If your pain level does not seem to decline in the expected time or if the relief is inadequate, call your health care team. Don't wait for your next scheduled appointment to report your situation. Your doctor may increase the dose of your pain medication or switch you to another medication or combination of medications.

In general, you should communicate any changes in your physical, emotional, and psychological condition after beginning pain medication. If pain medication doesn't work, make sure you inform your caregivers and a member of the health care team.

Communication and perseverance are crucial in making sure you receive the most effective combination and doses of pain medications.

The Pain Log

You may find it helpful to keep a record or diary to track the onset, duration, location, quality, patterns, and severity of pain you are experiencing.

Filling out a daily pain log allows you to bring an accurate history of your pain to your next meeting with your health care team. This can help them to monitor any trends in your pain as well as how well pain treatment is working for you. (Once you have begun treatment to relieve your pain, it will be helpful to complete a pain log that includes details about medicine dosages and effects; see page 103 of chapter 5.)

Assessment for Recurrence of Pain

Once your pain is under control, you and your caregivers must be watchful for signs of its return. Pain can reappear in an old location, but it is important to realize that new areas of the body may also become involved over time, and new pain may have a different quality from what you experienced in the past.

If you experience the onset of new pain, increased severity of existing pain, or side effects you suspect may be caused by pain medications or other treatments, do not hesitate to tell caregivers or contact your health care team. The more quickly you inform others about a change in your pain status, the more quickly steps can be taken to control pain and reduce side effects. There is no way of knowing whether the pain will go away on its own, and nothing will be gained by "waiting it out." Suffering in silence may seem noble and independent, but it is unnecessary and doesn't accomplish anything. In fact, new studies suggest that uncontrolled pain actually lowers the pain threshold and decreases your tolerance to pain. Pain can and should be treated whenever it causes discomfort or interferes with your life.

When to Notify Your Health Care Team about Pain

Call your doctor or nurse if:

- you experience any new or severe pain
- you are unable to take anything by mouth, including pain medication
- the pain causes you to cry out, become still, or double over
- you have any questions about how to take your medications or if new symptoms accompany your pain (such as inability to walk, eat, sleep, or urinate)
- you are unable to sleep because of pain
- you have decreased appetite because of pain
- you cry, feel upset, feel helpless, or feel depressed because of your pain
- you notice new areas of redness or swelling in an area of pain
- your prescribed pain medicines do not relieve the pain or do not relieve it for long enough

---

Pain Log

	Time the pain started	How long the pain lasted	Where you felt pain	What the pain felt like	What you were doing when you felt pain	How severe the pain was
Sunday						
Monday						
Tuesday						
Wednesday						
Thursday						
Friday						
Saturday						

CHAPTER 5

Pain Relief through Medication

Mary was admitted to the hospital unit where I worked. She had back pain and went to surgery for a ruptured disc. Instead of a disc problem, it turned out that Mary had a large malignant tumor wrapped around her spine. Following her surgery, Mary's doctor treated her back pain with meperidine (Demerol). Nonetheless, she still pointed to the crying face on the faces scale when asked how bad her pain was. Mary's pain was caused by the cancer pressing on the nerves in her back and not the surgery.

Mary's oncologist knew that even though Demerol was sometimes used to treat short-term surgical pain, it is not effective for chronic cancer pain. I watched the medical oncologist change her pain medicine and quickly increase the dose until Mary had some relief. Mary soon pointed not to the crying face on the faces scale, but to a frown with no tears. This told us that Mary's pain was beginning to be relieved.

After continued adjustment of her pain medicine and the addition of other medicines, Mary pointed to a face with no frown and no tears, then to what appeared to be a smile. As I continued to be involved in Mary's care, I began to realize that relieving Mary's pain was how we could help Mary the most."

— Terri, a cancer nurse

THE GOAL OF PAIN THERAPY IS STRAIGHTFORWARD: to avoid pain that can be prevented and to control pain that cannot, while limiting medication-related side effects. Cancer pain can be treated in a variety of ways, including by treating the cancer itself with surgery, chemotherapy, and radiation. But the use of pain-relief medicines, known as drug therapy, is the cornerstone of pain treatment. Drug therapy brings significant relief in most cases, regardless of a patient's age or whether pain is acute or chronic.

When their pain is treated, people with cancer are often able to resume normal activities and enjoy an improved quality of life. Many doctors place a great deal of importance on making sure a patient can sleep without pain; adequate sleep not only increases tolerance to pain, it also boosts energy levels during the day and improves overall well-being. It is also important to ensure that patients can be comfortable while awake and at rest.

Determining Pain Medication(s) Appropriate for You

As a rule, your health care team will match the type and amount of recommended pain medication (or combination of medications) to the severity of your pain. Important factors to consider are your previous experiences with pain, the success of any previous drug therapy for pain relief, the type of cancer treatment being used, and your doctor's familiarity with the medications. Your health care team will be guided in decisions about which drugs to prescribe and at what dosages and frequencies based on information about the severity and character of your pain, your ability to tolerate of pain, and the potential for medication-related side effects.

Medications used to relieve pain, called analgesics, act on various parts of the nervous system to relieve pain without causing loss of consciousness. Analgesics provide only temporary relief, which is why they must be taken regularly to effectively decrease or eliminate symptoms.

The sedative effects of many pain medications are enhanced by alcohol. *Keep in mind that alcohol and other medications may have dangerous effects on your body when combined with pain medications.* Combining alcohol with prescription pain medicines (such as opioids) and anti-inflammatory medications (such as ibuprofen) can be dangerous. Alcohol with even small doses of these medications may cause problems. *Some nonprescription medications, such as those for allergies, may also increase the sedative effects of opioids.*

Types of Medicines Used to Control Cancer Pain

Mild pain relievers, many of which do not require a prescription, are often used to relieve mild cancer-related pain. If pain gets worse, your doctor will most likely prescribe more potent medications. Often, medications are combined to enhance pain relief or to relieve medication-related side effects. The types of pain-relief medications available are described here.

Nonsteroidal Anti-Inflammatory Drugs (NSAIDs)

Nonsteroidal anti-inflammatory drugs (NSAIDs) are the mainstay of drug therapy for those with mild pain, but they are also likely to be used for people with moderate or severe pain. NSAIDs do their work outside of the central nervous system by stopping the actions of a chemical called prostaglandin. Some types of prostaglandins are responsible for causing pain. By slowing down the rate of prostaglandin production, NSAIDs reduce pain. NSAIDs also reduce inflammation and pain caused by inflammation.

What's in a Name?

When discussing drugs, remember that every medication has two names: the generic name, which describes the chemical content of the drug, and the brand name, the name under which the drug is sold. Typically, the brand name is capitalized while the generic name is written in all lowercase letters.

A single generic drug may be marketed under several brand names. For example, the generic drug aspirin is sold under numerous well-known brand names, such as Bayer and Ecotrin. The generic drug acetaminophen is probably best known by the brand name Tylenol, though it is also sold under other brand names. And the generic drug ibuprofen is marketed under several brand names, including Motrin, Advil, and Nuprin. The generic name of a drug is printed on the label of a brand-name medication.

Some generic drugs are sold without any brand names attached. For instance, you can purchase a bottle of generic ibuprofen or generic acetaminophen. Generic drugs typically cost less than brand-name products.

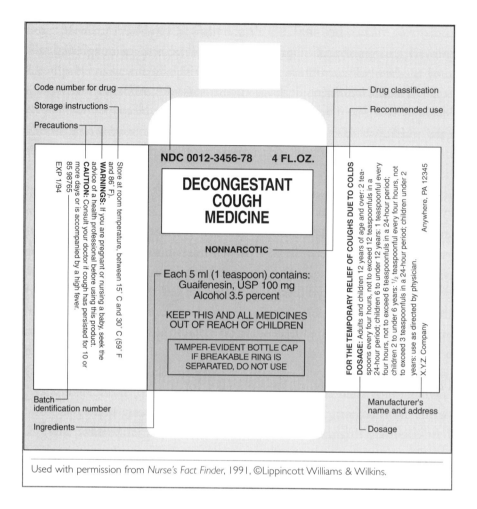

Code number for drug

Storage instructions

Precautions

Drug classification

Recommended use

NDC 0012-3456-78   4 FL.OZ.

DECONGESTANT COUGH MEDICINE

NONNARCOTIC

Each 5 ml (1 teaspoon) contains:
Guaifenesin, USP 100 mg
Alcohol 3.5 percent

KEEP THIS AND ALL MEDICINES
OUT OF REACH OF CHILDREN

TAMPER-EVIDENT BOTTLE CAP
IF BREAKABLE RING IS
SEPARATED, DO NOT USE

Store at room temperature, between 15° C and 30° C (59° F and 86° F).
WARNINGS: If you are pregnant or nursing a baby, seek the advice of a health professional before using this product.
CAUTION: Consult your doctor if cough has persisted for 10 or more days or is accompanied by a high fever.

85 98765
EXP 1/94

FOR THE TEMPORARY RELIEF OF COUGHS DUE TO COLDS
DOSAGE: Adults and children 12 years of age and over: 2 teaspoons every four hours, not to exceed 12 teaspoonfuls in a 24-hour period; children 6 to under 12 years: 1 teaspoonful every four hours, not to exceed 6 teaspoonfuls in a 24-hour period; children 2 to under 6 years: 1/2 teaspoonful every four hours, not to exceed 3 teaspoonfuls in a 24-hour period; children under 2 years: use as directed by physician.

X.Y.Z. Company   Anywhere, PA 12345

Batch
identification number

Ingredients

Manufacturer's
name and address

Dosage

There are about twenty different kinds of NSAIDs, including aspirin and ibuprofen (see *Appendix A*). Chemically, NSAIDs are similar, but the effectiveness of different medicines may vary. Some popular NSAIDs are widely advertised, such as those with the brand names Advil and Nuprin. Generic versions of the same products are often available at a lower price. Some NSAIDs that are available over-the-counter require a doctor's prescription at higher dose levels.

The cyclooxygenase-2 (COX-2) inhibitors are a newer type of NSAID often used to treat arthritis; they can help relieve cancer pain as well. COX-2 inhibitors such as celecoxib (Celebrex), rofecoxib (Vioxx), and valdecoxib (Bextra) are available by prescription only and are associated with fewer gastrointestinal side effects and bleeding problems than other NSAIDs.

If your doctor chooses an NSAID that is available without a prescription, it doesn't mean that the NSAID won't work to relieve your pain. NSAIDs can be surprisingly effective and are much stronger than many people realize. In many cases, NSAIDs successfully relieve cancer pain. This is especially true if patients "stay on top of the pain" by taking medicines on schedule rather than waiting to take them when the pain returns. It is easier to manage pain by taking the medicine on a regular schedule in the absence of pain than by waiting until the pain becomes troublesome.

The Most Effective NSAID for Your Situation

The first NSAID medication you take for pain control may not reduce your pain to an acceptable level. Keep a positive outlook; there are many drugs in the NSAID family your doctor can recommend. Finding out which one is most effective for you is often a matter of trial and error. Your doctor may first prescribe an NSAID that you remembered worked well in the past. The only way to know if one NSAID is more effective at relieving your current pain than another is to try it out and gauge the results.

NSAID Side Effects

Stomach upset and indigestion are the most common side effects of NSAIDs. Taking your medicines immediately following a meal with food or milk may reduce or prevent these side effects. NSAIDs can also cause vomiting, constipation, and bleeding in the stomach. If your stools are darker than normal or if you notice blood in your stool—both signs of bleeding in the gastrointestinal tract—tell your doctor or nurse. Be

> ### NSAIDs Aren't for Everyone
>
> In general, NSAIDs should be avoided by people who:
> - are allergic to aspirin
> - are on chemotherapy (anticancer drugs)
> - are on steroid medicines
> - have stomach ulcers or a history of ulcers, gout, or bleeding disorders
> - are taking prescription medicines for arthritis
> - are taking oral medicine for diabetes or gout
> - have kidney problems
> - will have surgery within a week
> - are taking blood-thinning medicine

careful not to mix NSAIDs with alcohol—taking NSAIDs and drinking alcohol can cause stomach upset and sometimes bleeding in the lining of the stomach.

Some people with bleeding or clotting disorders may not be able to take NSAIDs because of the effect of the medicines on the blood's ability to clot. People who are receiving chemotherapy drugs that can lower their level of blood platelets may be cautioned against taking NSAIDs during specific times of their chemotherapy cycle.

Other potential side effects of NSAIDs are dizziness, headache, ringing in the ears, fluid retention, dry mouth, and increased heart rate. NSAIDs may also produce stomach ulcers.

Each NSAID has a maximum dose that can be taken at one time. Higher doses produce no additional pain relief but increase the risk of side effects. You should take no more than the prescribed or recommended dose.

While receiving NSAIDs, you will be monitored closely for potential side effects. Elderly persons should be monitored carefully while taking NSAIDs. The long-term use of NSAIDs in older persons can lead to life-threatening risks of gastrointestinal bleeding.

Acetaminophen

Acetaminophen is a well-known nonopioid pain reliever that is effective against mild or moderate pain like an NSAID but does not reduce inflammation. The drug may be given alone or in a pill combined with a mild opioid (Tylenol III is one example).

Doses of acetaminophen should be limited to no more than four grams daily (equivalent to no more than eight extra-strength 500 mg tablets or 12 regular-strength 325 mg tablets). Some new studies indicate that older persons should take no more than two grams of acetaminophen in one day. Read medication labels carefully, and when calculating your daily dose, consider the acetaminophen you are receiving from all sources—including combination opioids and cold remedies, which may contain acetaminophen.

Acetaminophen Side Effects

Side effects associated with acetaminophen are rare. However, taking large doses daily for a long period of time or regularly drinking alcohol with the usual dose may cause liver or kidney damage.

If you are receiving chemotherapy, your doctor may ask that you not take acetaminophen regularly or that you not take it at specific times during your treatment. One of the side effects of many chemotherapy drugs is lowered white blood cell counts; this can result in infection. Your doctor will want to be able to watch for signs and symptoms of infection, and taking acetaminophen will mask the presence of a fever, which may be a sign of infection that requires immediate treatment.

Opioids

Opioids were once made from the opium poppy or poppy juice, but today most are synthetic, made by drug companies. (See *Appendix A* for detailed information on specific opioids and other pain-relief medicines.)

Opioids are exceedingly effective in relieving cancer pain. Unfortunately, opioids are sometimes wrongly associated with illegal "street" drugs. Furthermore, myths and misunderstandings have led to the underuse of opioids in many cases where people in significant pain would greatly benefit from them. Increasingly—in large part because of the experience gained from the hospice movement in England—health care professionals are recognizing the benefits of opioid analgesics for treating cancer pain.

Opioids can be given alone but are often prescribed in combination with nonopioid analgesics (i.e., NSAIDs or acetaminophen) as well as with other adjuvant medications (medications taken with pain relievers to enhance their effects). Opioids are usually given by mouth, but for patients who have difficulty swallowing or who have significant side effects when they take opioids by mouth, these drugs can also be given intravenously (into a vein), as rectal suppositories, or through a number of other drug delivery systems (see pages 89–93). Opioids are available in both short-acting and time-release forms with effects that may last for many hours.

Opioid Side Effects

You may experience mild side effects when taking opioid medications (see chapter 8 for more information about side effects and coping with them). The most common side effects are predictable and can usually be managed by either altering the dose or prescribing other medications to control the side effects. Typical side effects include sedation (drowsiness), constipation, nausea, and vomiting. Some people may also experience dizziness, mental effects (nightmares, confusion, or hallucinations), decreased rate and depth of breathing, difficulty in urinating, or itching. See *If You Have a Reaction to Pain Medicine* on this page for information about side effects you should report to your doctor right away.

Mild Opioids

If nonopioid analgesics do not bring sufficient pain relief within 24 to 48 hours, your doctor is likely to add a mild opioid to your treatment regimen. Codeine is one example of a mild opioid. Many people who take opioids benefit from continuing to take regular doses of NSAIDs or acetaminophen.

Because the two types of drugs attack pain in distinct ways, combining them often enhances pain relief. NSAIDs cut off the pain signal at the site of pain, while opioids block the signals passing through the central nervous system and decrease the sensitivity of pain receptors.

For many patients, mild opioids in combination with NSAIDs can prevent or control pain. The dose of mild opioids is increased

---

If You Have a Reaction to Pain Medicine

Serious pain medicine side effects are rare. However, some people may have serious reactions to pain medicines. Call the doctor or nurse immediately if you experience any of the following symptoms when taking pain medicines, and alert your caregivers to these signs that you may be having a serious reaction:

- hallucinations
- ringing or buzzing in the ears
- confusion or being "out of it"
- great trouble waking up even when others try to wake you
- severe trembling, uncontrolled muscle movements, or convulsions (seizures)
- inability to hold in urine or stool when this was not a problem in the past
- nausea or vomiting with no relief
- hives, itching, skin rash, or swelling of the face
- anxiousness or feeling "fidgety"
- slow breathing (fewer than eight breaths per minute) or very shallow breathing (short breaths that don't take in much air)

until adequate pain relief is achieved. As with NSAIDs, finding the most effective opioid pain reliever is often a matter of trial and error.

Strong Opioids

If pain becomes severe and does not respond to mild opioids, stronger opioids may be needed. Strong opioids are the most powerful and most effective pain relievers. The best known strong opioid is morphine. Morphine is frequently the first choice for treating severe cancer-related pain. A number of brand-name drugs contain morphine or morphine-like chemicals (MS Contin, Oramorph). Other frequently used strong opioids include hydromorphone (Dilaudid), levorphanol (Levo-Dromoran), methadone (Dolophine, Methadose), and oxycodone (OxyContin). Your doctor is likely to continue to prescribe NSAIDs and adjuvant medication along with a strong opioid.

Some opioid pain medicines, such as oxycodone (OxyContin) and morphine or morphine-like products (MS Contin, Oramorph), are available in "sustained release" (long-acting) forms that last for eight or twelve hours. Kadian is a slow-release morphine pill that lasts for up to 24 hours; fentanyl is available as a topical medicine in the form of a patch that delivers the analgesic continuously through the skin for 72 hours; and fentanyl (Actiq) is also available in a transmucosal (absorbed through the lining of the mouth) form.

Treatment with strong opioids begins at low doses under careful medical observation. The dose is raised until pain relief is achieved or until side effects become a problem. If one drug is not effective or if a person is particularly sensitive to its side effects, your doctor may try another drug. The new drug will probably be prescribed at a dose equivalent to that of the last opioid, since you will have already had time to adjust to the effects of opioids in general.

Although it was once believed that strong opioids were not very effective when given by mouth, today the oral route is preferred. Morphine and other strong opioids given orally appear to work extremely well at all dose levels, though other routes of administration are necessary for some patients.

Doctors carefully adjust the doses of opioids so there is little possibility of overdose. Therefore, it is important that two different doctors do not prescribe opioids for you unless they first talk with each other.

Tell any doctors you deal with if you drink alcohol or take tranquilizers, sleeping aids, antidepressants, antihistamines, or any other medicines that make you sleepy. Combining opioids with these substances can be dangerous, even at low doses, and can lead to an overdose with symptoms of weakness, difficulty in breathing, confusion, anxiety, and severe drowsiness or dizziness.

Other Types of Pain Medications

Adjuvant Medicines

Medicines to enhance the effects of NSAIDs or opioids may be prescribed along with analgesics. These adjuvant medicines (medicines given along with a primary treatment) are typically used to treat other illnesses but may be used along with a primary cancer pain medicine. Antidepressants, anticonvulsants, and corticosteroids are a few examples. Though some research shows a few adjuvant drugs possess pain-relieving qualities (these are called adjuvant analgesics), adjuvant medicines are rarely used alone for pain control.

The table on the next page offers an overview of the major classes of adjuvant medicines that might be prescribed to enhance pain relief. (See *Appendix A* for more detailed information about specific medications.)

Anesthetic Treatments

Anesthetic techniques, such as nerve blocks, are used to treat cancer pain that is not relieved by other techniques (see chapter 6 for more information about nerve blocks). For example, neuropathic pain—tingling and burning sensations or weakness or numbness in your hands and feet—caused by the invasion of or compression of a nerve may not be easily relieved by pain medicines taken by mouth.

Most anesthesia techniques block nerves. For example, pain in the chest wall and abdominal wall can be relieved by interrupting the nerves that exit from the spinal cord to supply these sites. Pain in the legs, groin, and lower back can be helped by injecting drugs into the spaces around the spine to numb the nerves that receive pain signals from these sites. Patients with

Adjuvant Medicines

Drug Class	Generic Name	Trade Name	Action	Potential Side Effects
Muscle relaxants/ Antianxiety drugs	diazepam alprazolam lorazepam haloperidol	Valium Xanax Ativan Haldol	· Used to treat anxiety. · Also used to treat muscle spasms that may cause severe pain.	· Drowsiness. · May cause urinary incontinence.
Anticonvulsants	carbamazepine clonazepam gabapentin phenytoin	Tegretol Klonopin Neurontin Dilantin	· Helps to control tingling or burning from nerve injury caused by the cancer or cancer therapy.	· Liver problems and lowered number of red and white blood cells. · Gabapentin may cause sedation and dizziness.
Antidepressants: tricyclic	amitriptyline hydrochloride imipramine nortriptyline desipramine doxepin	Elavil Tofranil Aventyl HCl, Pamelor Norpramin Sinequan	· Used to treat tingling or burning pain from damaged nerves. · Nerve injury can result from surgery, radiation therapy, or chemotherapy.	· Dry mouth, sleepiness, constipation, drop in blood pressure with dizziness or fainting when standing. · Blurred vision. · Urinary retention. · Patients with heart disease may have an irregular heartbeat.
Antidepressants: selective serotonin reuptake inhibitors	sertraline fluoxetine paroxetine	Zoloft Prozac Paxil	· May be used to treat depression in those with pain, but not used to treat pain itself.	· Nausea, dizziness, dry mouth, sexual dysfunction, insomnia, diarrhea, tremors, drowsiness.
Corticosteroids	dexamethasone prednisone	Decadron Prednisone	· Helps relieve bone pain, pain caused by spinal cord and brain tumors, and pain caused by inflammation. · Increases appetite. · Relieves nausea associated with chemotherapy.	· Fluid buildup in the body. · Increased blood sugar. · Stomach irritation. · Sleeplessness. · Mood changes.

upper abdominal pain from pancreatic cancer can get good relief from interruption of the nerves near the pancreas.

Both opioid medicines and local anesthetics are used for this method of pain relief. Morphine and fentanyl are the medicines used most commonly for intrathecal administration. A combination of opioids and anesthetic agents, such as bupivacaine and ropivacaine, are used especially in patients who have not received adequate relief with opioids alone.

A continuous epidural infusion is used when the pain is difficult to treat, as in cases of advanced metastatic disease involving the pelvis and lower body. An infusion pump may deliver the pain medicine to the spinal column through a catheter, or a small reservoir may be surgically implanted in the body to dispense the drug in small doses over time. The advantage of this method is that it provides effective relief without disrupting the function of the muscles and nerves.

Side effects from medicines given into the spine may include urinary retention, itching, nausea, vomiting, and decreased respirations.

Another anesthetic technique used to help relieve pain involves the use of local anesthetics such as xylocaine. Examples include swabbing a topical anesthetic on a painful mouth sore or applying it to the skin before inserting an IV catheter. Local anesthetics are effective in helping relieve pain on the surface of the skin or a superficial area of pain.

Anticonvulsants

Anticonvulsants (antiseizure medicines), such as gabapentin (Neurontin), carbamazepine (Tegretol), phenytoin (Dilantin), and clonazepam (Klonopin), are used primarily to control convulsions (e.g., seizures associated with epilepsy). But as adjuvant medicines, they may also relieve sharp stabbing, shooting, burning, or tingling pain caused by tumors pressing on nerves, especially in the head and neck. Such pain can be difficult to treat with opioids alone. Anticonvulsants are occasionally prescribed to reduce pain following surgery and for people with limb amputation, stump pain, or pain in the lower extremities. Gabapentin, the most commonly used anticonvulsant, has a wide dose range. It may cause side effects such as sleepiness, dizziness, and fatigue. Call your doctor or nurse right away if you have difficulty walking, difficulty urinating, a rash, changes in vision, or any problems taking the drug.

Antidepressants

Some standard (tricyclic) antidepressants may be used to relieve tingling and burning pain. For example, amitryptyline (Elavil, Endep), doxepin (Sinequan), and imipramine (Tofranil) may reduce neuropathic pain, a dull, burning sensation caused when cancer cells invade or press on nerves. Taking regular doses for up to two weeks may be necessary before neuropathic pain is relieved.

Tricyclic antidepressants have also been used to control pain caused by mastectomy and other surgeries. The most notable side effects associated with tricyclic antidepressants include dry mouth, constipation, low blood pressure, and sedation, all of which can be troublesome for patients using opioids.

More recently developed antidepressants (i.e., selective serotonin reuptake inhibitors, such as fluoxetine [Prozac], paroxetine [Paxil], and sertraline [Zoloft]) may also be used to reduce depression experienced by many people who live with pain, but they are not used to treat pain directly.

Corticosteroids

Corticosteroids (also called steroids) reduce swelling, inflammation, and pain caused by tumors that press on or invade nerves or bones. Steroids also can promote appetite and improve mood. The drug dexamethasone (Decadron) is commonly used to treat back pain due to spinal cord compression. Prednisone (Deltasone) is a common choice for treating patients who have advanced cancer. People with advanced cancer who receive steroids often need lower doses of opioids to control pain. Corticosteroids may also be used as a treatment for certain cancers.

Steroids can cause a number of undesirable and potentially dangerous side effects, such as adrenal insufficiency, which is characterized by loss of appetite, nausea, dizziness, depression, low blood sugar, and low blood pressure. Adrenal insufficiency can be fatal. It can also cause fluid retention which can lead to high blood pressure and heart failure, low calcium, low potassium, osteoporosis, and increased susceptibility to infections and delay in healing. Because of these risks, corticosteroids are often prescribed for short-term use to control flare-ups of acute pain. Keep in mind that it may be safer for elderly persons to use steroids and low-dose long-acting opioids rather than long-term NSAID therapy.

Muscle Relaxant/Antianxiety Agents

Cancer patients commonly become anxious during exams and treatment. Severe anxiety can interfere with a person's ability to function, decrease their ability to comprehend, and increase painful sensations. When anxiety is linked directly to pain, a pain-relief medicine may reduce both.

Antianxiety drugs, such as mild tranquilizers, do not relieve pain directly but help muscles relax, can help people feel calmer, and may counter the anxiety-producing effects of some pain medications. Tranquilizers are also prescribed for people who experience panic attacks. Patients who don't respond to tranquilizers may require antipsychotic medications such as haloperidol (Haldol), which may reduce confusion and agitation.

Side effects of tranquilizers include drowsiness, confusion, and uncoordinated movements. Patients using tranquilizers should avoid alcohol, because the combination of the two can lead to extremely dangerous side effects.

Methods Used for Drug Delivery

Most pain medicines are taken by mouth, usually as tablets, capsules, liquids, or gelcaps. They are typically taken with a large glass of water or other liquid unless the doctor advises otherwise. Do not take your medicine with alcoholic beverages.

Oral medications may cause problems for patients who have difficulty swallowing, or they may cause side effects such as nausea and vomiting. In such cases, your doctor may administer the medicine in a different way, such as through a skin patch, suppository, or by injection under the skin.

During the course of an illness, most people need to take pain medications by multiple methods. This is important because the way drugs are administered can make a big difference in their effectiveness. For example, medications given orally or rectally may take longer to work, but they may last longer than medications given intravenously.

Oral

As a rule, chronic pain is best treated orally. Compared with other drug delivery methods, the oral route is the easiest, least expensive, and safest. Orally administered drugs generally provide the longest relief. Oral medications also allow people to be more active by freeing them from relying on tubes and pumps that hinder mobility. Drugs taken orally are generally given in higher doses than those given by other means because the drug must pass through the stomach's acidic environment before being absorbed into the bloodstream. Patients must remember to take the correct doses of these medications and to take them on schedule.

For patients who cannot eat solid foods or have trouble swallowing pills, some pain medicines are available in liquid form, which may easier to ingest. Some opioids, including morphine, are available in high-concentration forms, which can be given in very small volumes.

Transmucosal

When a patient cannot swallow tablets or liquid, some medications can be put inside the cheek or between the cheek and gums and absorbed (for example, transmucosal fentanyl [ACTIQ], which is used to treat breakthrough pain). This route of administration is called transmucosal, meaning that the medicine is absorbed through the mucous lining of the mouth. This is also a favored method for people who have difficulty swallowing. However, bitter flavors, irritation, and poor absorption can limit their usefulness.

Sublingual

Other medications are taken by putting the drug under the tongue for absorption. This route of administration is called sublingual. This method can be used for patients who are unable to take oral medicines. Many hospices give liquid morphine this way to patients who cannot swallow.

Transdermal (Skin Patch)

The transdermal method of drug delivery uses a bandage-like skin patch that releases medicine through the skin and into the bloodstream. The medicine enters the body slowly and steadily for up to 72 hours and allows for flexible dosing. Transdermal administration is particularly useful for patients who are already taking strong opioids but are unable to swallow them, who may experience nausea and vomiting after chemotherapy, or who have a blockage in their intestines. Skin patches are usually placed on the chest or back. Older persons or those who have lost large amounts of subcutaneous tissue because of weight loss may not absorb medication well through the transdermal route and should be monitored carefully for pain control.

Getting to the right dose using this method of administration takes some time. The maximum dose is limited. Another fast-acting medicine is often required to treat breakthrough pain. The patch is not suitable for those needing quick dose changes. The patch may need to be changed every 48 hours.

Rectal Suppositories

Rectal suppositories are often used when a person cannot swallow pills, experiences nausea and vomiting after taking pain medications orally, or is unable to eat or drink before surgery. Once placed in the rectum, a suppository melts and releases the drug into the body. The process is painless and generally causes only minimal discomfort for most people. Opioids and nonopioids are available as suppositories. Suppositories can also be placed through abdominal openings (called stomas) made during surgery for colorectal cancer.

This is a simple, safe method. However, suppositories must be avoided if there are sores in or around the rectum. They cannot be used if a patient has diarrhea or hemorrhoids. Some elderly or disabled people might need assistance using suppositories. Suppositories are also relatively expensive.

Many people with cancer and their families simply don't like administering medications rectally and use suppositories only if oral pain relief is not available.

Injections

Intravenous (IV) Injections and Intravenous Lines

With intravenous injections, drugs are delivered through a needle or thin plastic catheter that has been placed directly into large veins in the arm and remains there. When IV lines are inserted into large arm veins, they are called Hickmans, Broviacs, or peripherally inserted central catheters (PICC lines).

Both IV injections and infusions are suitable for patients who have constant nausea and vomiting, cannot swallow, have mouth and throat pain, and are confused or have mental status changes that prohibit swallowing medicines. They are also useful for delivering very high doses of medication or when dose changes are needed quickly and are made often. They provide a constant and rapid onset of pain relief. With IV lines, patients do not require an injection every time drugs are given. The IV tubing protrudes from the skin a few inches and dressings are changed as needed.

Implanted ports are a new way to deliver medicine into a large vein in the chest. These circular, metal ports are about one inch wide and one inch deep. Ports are usually surgically placed under the skin of the upper chest. A nurse locates its exact placement by gently pushing on the skin and feeling the small round disc where the medicine is to be injected into the port. The nurse cleans the skin with a solution and injects medicine into the port, which flows into the vein. This method provides easy IV access without frequent injections into a vein. There is some risk of infection, so this route is used only when less invasive methods are not available.

Subcutaneous (SQ or SC) Injection and Infusion

With subcutaneous infusion, a small needle is implanted just under the skin. Every few hours, the patient or a caregiver can give medicines manually through tubing connected to the implanted needle. Alternatively, an automated pump can be hooked directly to the implanted needle to inject medication on a preset schedule. With this delivery method, patients do not have to receive an injection every time medication is needed.

Intraspinal Injections

With this method, drugs are injected either into the epidural space, which is the space between the bones of the spine and the outer layer of the spinal cord, or into the intrathecal space of the spinal canal, which is the space just outside the spinal cord. Opioids are more potent when given into the intrathecal space as compared to the epidural space.

Intraspinal injections are used when the patient's cancer pain is responsive to opioids but when the side effects are too great to be tolerated when given IV or by mouth. When given directly into the central nervous system, the medicines do not affect the entire body, so there are fewer side effects.

Intramuscular (IM) Injection

Some pain medications can be injected directly into the muscle tissue with a syringe, but this route is not recommended. It is difficult to predict how long the intramuscularly (IM) injected medicines will be effective, and the injections are painful. Subcutaneous injections are less painful, and medications administered subcutaneously are absorbed as well as those that are injected into the muscle.

Patient-Controlled Analgesia (PCA)

One of the newer approaches to cancer pain management allows patients to control the administration of medicines at a rate and dosage that they choose. This method is referred to as patient-controlled analgesia, or PCA. It may be used by patients at home and is very common in many cancer care facilities.

PCA (sometimes called self-administered analgesia) uses an electronic infusion pump attached to a drug reservoir and a timing device. A tube is connected to a small needle or thin plastic catheter inserted under the skin (SQ) or into a vein (IV). When patients feel pain, they press a button on the pump and receive a preset dose of medication. The timer is adjustable so that no more than a certain amount of drug can be taken over a given time. PCA is often used after surgery or for anyone with severe pain.

Some studies suggest that patients who control their own medication tend to be discharged earlier after surgery and may suffer fewer chronic pain problems later. Patients who control pain themselves may use lower total doses of medications than would have been prescribed by doctors. Most people prefer this arrangement to receiving injections every few hours. If nothing else, PCA offers a psychological advantage, because pain is often easier to bear if you know you can relieve it whenever you want.

Today, miniature pumps are available that fit into a fanny pack, backpack, or purse, and deliver a continuous infusion of analgesic medication.

Managing Your Drug Therapy Program

The most effective way to control pain with drugs is to keep symptoms at bay and prevent them from returning. For this reason, it is important for you to closely follow your medication schedules, even if you are not in pain, and pay attention to when it is time to take the next dose. Once pain reemerges, it becomes much more difficult to control. Following your doctor's directions about when and how much medication you take is important to the success of your drug therapy program. Get in the habit of regularly informing your doctor or another member of your health care team about how well your medications are working so that your therapy can be altered if necessary.

A person who requires a high dose of an opioid for a long time to relieve pain is likely to become physically dependent on it. Physical dependence is not addiction. Addiction is psychological dependence—taking a drug for psychological effects, not for relief of pain. A person who is physically dependent on opioids might experience withdrawal symptoms if he or she suddenly stopped taking the medication.

Ideally, drug therapy will relieve your pain without causing undue side effects, but sometimes these two goals must be weighed against each other. If you need to be taken off opioid medications, your doctor will advise gradually cutting back to minimize the uncomfortable symptoms of withdrawal, which may include flu-like symptoms, agitation, sleeplessness, fear, worsening of pain, and excessive perspiration. Tell your doctor immediately if you experience any of these symptoms. They can be treated and tend to disappear within a few days or a few weeks, but it is best to avoid withdrawal altogether by decreasing the dose of opioids slowly.

Controlling Breakthrough Pain

It is common for people with persistent pain to experience episodes of breakthrough pain, a brief and often severe flare of pain that occurs even though a person may be taking pain medicine regularly for persistent pain (see chapter 1 for more information about types of pain). If you have breakthrough pain, it does not mean that the pain medicine you are using regularly is not working well; breakthrough pain may occur even when you are taking the correct dose of pain medicine on a regular schedule for persistent pain.

Medicines Used for Breakthrough Pain

Breakthrough pain is best treated with medicines that work quickly and for short periods of time. Breakthrough medicines are usually given on an as-needed basis, which means that they are taken when you are feeling breakthrough pain. Because these short-acting medicines (sometimes called "rescue" medicines) work faster than the medicines you are using for your persistent pain, you can get pain relief sooner. They also stay in your body for a shorter period of time, so they cause fewer side effects.

The most common medicine used to treat breakthrough pain is immediate-release morphine given as tablets, capsules, or liquid. Other medicines for breakthrough pain that promise faster and more effective pain relief are currently being developed. Ask your doctor or nurse about your treatment options for breakthrough pain.

How to Take Medicines for Breakthrough Pain

It is important that you take short-acting medicine when you first begin to feel breakthrough pain so it can begin to work to relieve the pain. Do not let the pain build up and become harder to control. You may also want to take a dose of your breakthrough medicine if you know that you are likely to have breakthrough pain with a particular activity. Follow the directions given to you. If the labeled dose does not relieve your breakthrough pain or if you think you are having too many episodes of breakthrough pain, contact your doctor or nurse. They may need to adjust the dose or frequency of your breakthrough pain medicine.

There may be times when you experience breakthrough pain right before or after taking your persistent pain medicine. At these times, you should take your breakthrough pain medicine and continue to take your persistent pain medicine according to the directions given to you by your doctor or nurse. It may be helpful to mark your medicine bottles clearly "for breakthrough pain" or "for regular pain." If you find that you are regularly having breakthrough pain right before your usual dose of persistent pain medicine, talk to your doctor or nurse. They may need to adjust the dose or the frequency of your persistent pain medicine.

Taking two different opioid pain medicines will not cause more side effects. In fact, both a long-acting and a short-acting medicine are given so that you will have fewer side effects. Most people only have breakthrough pain a few times a day, and the breakthrough pain is usually much more severe than their persistent pain. By taking a short-acting medicine for breakthrough pain, you are getting the extra medicine when

When to Notify Your Doctor

If you have chronic cancer pain and are taking medicines to control your pain, call the doctor or nurse immediately if any of the following conditions exist:

- you experience any new or severe pain
- you are unable to take anything by mouth, including pain medication
- your prescribed pain medicines do not relieve the pain or do not relieve it for long enough
- you become constipated, nauseated, or confused
- you have any questions about how to take your medications or if new symptoms accompany your pain (such as inability to walk, eat, sleep, or urinate)
- you are unable to sleep because of pain
- you become so groggy that it's difficult to carry on a conversation or stay awake
- you cry, feel upset, feel helpless, or feel depressed because of your pain
- you experience hallucinations (see things that aren't actually there)
- you feel disoriented
- you are unwilling to move, or muscles are very tense when moving
- the pain is constant, remains in one spot, or gets stronger
- the pain causes you to cry out, become still, or double over
- you notice new redness, swelling, or pus
- you get hives, itches, or a rash
- you experience uncontrolled muscle movements (twitches or jerks)
- you have decreased appetite because of pain
- pain continues to be a problem in between doses of long-acting medicines
- pain interferes with your normal activities, such as eating, sleeping, working, and sexual activity

you need it. Generally, you can expect the same types of side effects from your breakthrough pain medicines as from your long-acting medicines.

If your breakthrough pain medicine is not relieving your breakthrough pain, if you are having breakthrough pain more than two times a day, or if you have any questions about when to take your persistent pain or breakthrough pain medicines, contact your doctor or nurse.

Tolerance, Dependence, and Addiction

Many people worry that they will get "hooked" on opioids and won't be able to stop taking them. This is one of the greatest misconceptions about opioids and one that often results in the underuse of pain medications. Patients who take opioids to relieve pain are not addicts, nor are they at serious risk of becoming addicts, no matter how much of the drug they take or how often they take it. Opioids are powerful drugs that should be used only under a doctor's supervision, but the fear of addiction is unfounded. Yet many people with cancer still fear opioids and some health care professionals resist prescribing them, even when they are most needed.

Drug Tolerance

In most cases, when a drug dose and schedule that manages pain has been established, you can continue to follow it unless the disease worsens or other pain occurs. Sometimes people develop drug tolerance: their bodies adjust to the medication so that it does not relieve pain as effectively as it once did. Notify your doctor if your drug dosage is no longer working so he or she can increase the drug dose or suggest a different opioid medication. *Increased opioid doses do not lead to dependence or addiction.* A pain assessment will help your doctor determine the cause of increasing pain.

Many doctor, nurses, and patients still do not understand that tolerance differs from addiction. The two are completely different and should not be confused. Yet misinformation about opioids leads some health care professionals to limit or stop their use when they notice a patient is becoming drug tolerant. Some believe that if "too much" of a drug is used now, the medication will not work later when the patient "really needs it." This assumption is incorrect. People in pain may benefit from opioids at any given point during their pain experience.

The Myths about Opioids

Misunderstanding the facts about opioids may prevent patients and health care teams from employing opioids to treat pain. The following are common opioid myths:

- **"Opioids pose a strong risk of addiction."** False. The risk of addiction is less than one in 3,000. Unfortunately, the misplaced fear of addiction often means that these drugs are not used as frequently as they should be—or in the right doses—to provide adequate pain relief.
- **"Opioids produce euphoria, which inevitably leads to being hooked."** Not true. People taking opioids for pain relief seldom report feeling euphoric. Even if they do, it is unlikely that they will continue to seek drugs for their euphoric effects after the pain has abated.
- **"People are given morphine only when they're at death's door."** False. In good cancer management, opioids are administered as soon as pain becomes moderately severe. Opioids are appropriate treatment when nonopioids alone fail to provide the amount and duraton of relief the person needs.
- **"Morphine doesn't work when taken by mouth."** False. This belief originated from some faulty studies done some years ago. In fact, oral morphine is very effective. (However, injected opioids may work faster at lower doses.)
- **"People always need high doses of opioids."** False. Every person is different. Most people require only moderate doses; in fact many people with advanced cancer and chronic severe pain need no more than 20 mg every four hours, no matter how long the therapy lasts.
- **"I'll die of an overdose."** Many people fear opioids because of news reports about drug users who die of overdoses. Even though the doses required for adequate pain relief are sometimes high, they are rarely if ever large enough to cause death. Among substance abusers, death usually results when they take outrageously high doses or consume dangerous combinations of substances. And addicts often take illegal opioids manufactured by amateurs, compounds that contain impurities or are "cut" with other substances such as talcum powder.
- **"There's a limit to the effective dose of an opioid."** Not so. The stronger the pain is, the more is required for relief. NSAIDs do have a ceiling dose (as does acetaminophen), but opioids can be used in increasing amounts until they bring the pain under control. Furthermore, increasing the dose (often a necessary step in managing the pain of progressive cancer) does not increase the already minimal risk of addiction.
- **"People taking opioids always need to take antinausea drugs."** Some do, especially in the beginning. Women are more prone to feeling nausea and vomiting from opioids. But in most cases, antinausea therapy can be stopped after a few days.
- **"People should take morphine only when they feel the need."** Not true. The best strategy is to take regular doses around the clock, rather than on an as-needed basis.

Drug Dependence

There are two kinds of drug dependence: physical dependence and psychological dependence. Neither is the same as drug tolerance. *Physical dependence* is normal and predictable, and it is not a very serious result of using opioids. Anyone who takes a high enough dose of an opioid for a long enough time is likely to become physically dependent on it. The most obvious signs of dependency are withdrawal symptoms that appear when a person suddenly stops taking a drug. Withdrawal symptoms may include agitation, fear, chills, sweating, shaking, sleeplessness, and worsening pain. Though withdrawal is an unpleasant experience, it can easily be avoided and managed if opioid doses are reduced gradually over time. Physical dependence is *not* addiction.

Psychological Dependence and Addiction

When trained health professionals refer to addiction, they mean *psychological dependence*. Addicts take drugs to satisfy physical, emotional, and psychological needs, not to treat medical problems. An addict's life is centered around obtaining and taking drugs, despite financial, legal, or health consequences. Using an opioid is only one potential factor in developing a psychological dependence. Other important variables include a person's social, economic, and psychiatric background.

Pain is often not adequately treated because of the fear that increased use of opioids can lead to abuse. Though it is possible for patients who take opioids for pain to become psychologically addicted, the risk is incredibly small, especially among patients with no history of substance abuse.

Changing Your Pain Medicine or Drug Therapy Plan

If one medicine or treatment does not work, there is almost always another one that you can try. If your medication schedule or the method by which you are taking medicine does not work for you, changes can be made. Talk to your doctor or nurse about finding the pain medicine or method that works best for you. You may need a different pain medicine, a combination of pain medicines, or a change in the dose of your pain medicines if any of the following are true:

- your pain is not relieved
- your pain medicine does not start working within the time your doctor said it would
- your pain medicine does not work for the length of time your doctor said it would
- you have breakthrough pain
- you experience serious side effects such as trouble breathing, dizziness, and rashes; call your doctor right away if these occur. Side effects such as sleepiness, nausea, and itching usually go away after your body adjusts to the medication. Let your doctor know if these bother you.
- the schedule or the way you are taking the medicine does not work for you

In addition to changing medications, your doctor can choose other strategies to improve your pain treatment. He or she might look into the following changes to your pain-relief plan:

- Increase the dose of medicine. Sometimes there is not enough medicine in the body to prevent pain. If so, your doctor may increase the dose until adequate pain relief is achieved.
- Shorten time between doses. The right amount of pain medication may not remain in the bloodstream to alleviate pain because the drug isn't being taken often enough. If so, your doctor may shorten the time between doses. You can help to determine if this is a problem by writing down the time you take pain medication and how much time passes before the pain returns.
- Suggest short-acting or immediate-release opioids for breakthrough pain. If you experience breakthrough pain while taking your regular, long-acting pain medicines as prescribed, your doctor can prescribe special doses of pain relievers that work very quickly. Sometimes people need to have their dose of pain relievers almost doubled to prevent breakthrough pain from happening again.

- Prescribe a medication in a different form or with a different delivery technique. In addition to being given by mouth, medicines can be administered in a number of other ways, such as into a vein, through a skin patch, and through a rectal suppository.
- Use radiation therapy. Sometimes radiation therapy is prescribed to shrink a tumor that is causing pain (see chapter 6 for more information).
- Refer you to a pain clinic. Universities and large hospitals have special clinics to evaluate and treat chronic pain. Pain clinic staff members are specially trained to manage pain using a variety of techniques, including nerve blocks that stop the pain for a short time until other methods are prescribed. Most pain clinics require a doctor's referral.

Pain Records, Charts, and Logs

To treat pain optimally, it is important to gather as much information as possible during pain treatment. If people do not write down their experiences, most have trouble remembering in detail when they experience pain, the nature of the pain at any particular time, what they did to treat it, or what they were doing when it occurred.

In chapter 4, the pain log introduced for use prior to pain-relief treatment helped track the time of pain onset and its duration, location, quality, triggers, and severity. Keeping a pain log during pain treatment allows you to document pain and actions taken to relieve it, including drug therapy. Ideally, a daily pain log not only tracks pain levels, but also helps patients, caregivers, and medical staff members understand the effects pain and pain medications have on you, what steps work best to ease your pain, and the best times of day to take pain medications. A pain log can also indicate whether certain physical activities are closely associated with pain and need to be curtailed. Sometimes a pain log indicates clear patterns of improvement after only a few days of regular recording.

What to Include in a Pain Record

Details that you may want to track in a pain log include:

- a pain rating scale that describes your pain before and after using a pain-relief medicine (see chapter 4 for more information about pain rating scales)
- the name and dose of the pain medicine you take
- how long the pain medicine works
- the time you take pain medicine
- any activity that seems to be affected by the pain or that increases or decreases the pain
- any activity that you cannot engage in because of the pain
- any pain-relief methods used, other than medicine, such as rest, relaxation techniques, distraction, meditation, or imagery

By tracking the particular time of day you felt pain, the medication you took for it, any nondrug techniques you tried, and your emotional state, you will be able to more clearly convey your particular pain control needs to your doctor, nurse, or caregiver. The following page shows a sample pain log that may be used to track your pain throughout the day.

Pain and Pain-Relief Measures Record

Time	Severity from 0 (no pain) to 10 (severe)	Description of how pain feels	What you were doing when it began (e.g., walking, sleeping)	Name and amount of medication taken	Nondrug techniques you tried	Pain Relief (pain severity on a scale of 0 to 10)
Midnight						
1 a.m.						
2 a.m.						
3 a.m.						
4 a.m						
5 a.m.						
6 a.m.						
7 a.m.						
8 a.m.						
9 a.m.						
10 a.m.						
11 a.m.						
12 p.m.						
1 p.m.						
2 p.m.						
3 p.m.						
4 p.m.						
5 p.m.						
6 p.m.						
7 p.m.						
8 p.m.						
9 p.m.						
10 p.m.						
11 p.m.						

CHAPTER 6

Other Medical Approaches to Pain Management

Bruce was 68 years old when he began having abdominal pains and noticed the whites of his eyes taking on a yellowish hue. After several tests at the doctor's office and the local hospital, he was diagnosed with pancreatic cancer. A CT scan showed that part of his pancreas was pushing against his small intestine and several large tumors were present in his liver and in other parts of his abdomen. He was started on oral morphine to control his pain but was still uncomfortable even when other pain medications were added.

ORAL PAIN MEDICATION IS THE SIMPLEST, least invasive, most versatile, and often most effective method of relieving cancer-related pain. In most cases, patients experience significant pain relief from one or more oral analgesic medications. Of course, treating the cancer itself is an important way to relieve pain and other symptoms of cancer.

However, even after many attempts to determine the most effective analgesic combinations and dosages, medications may not adequately relieve pain or may cause intolerable side effects. When analgesic therapy fails to relieve pain adequately, doctors may turn to more invasive and complex methods of pain control.

Palliative Therapy for Pain Control

The three most commonly used primary cancer therapies are radiation therapy, surgery, and chemotherapy. Primary therapies are those directed against cancer (which may be the cause of pain). Each method may be used alone or in combination with another in an attempt to: (1) cure the cancer; (2) control the cancer or make the cancer go away for a while; or (3) treat the cancer in order to control or relieve symptoms caused by the cancer.

When cancer treatment is used to relieve pain, increase comfort, and improve quality of life, it is called palliative therapy. Doctors can help relieve cancer symptoms, such as pain, by using some form of palliative therapy. In addition to the three types of therapy listed above, hormonal therapy and treatment with bisphosphonates (drugs that slow down the action of bone-eating cells called osteoclasts, thereby slowing the spread of cancer in the bones) may also be used to palliate, or help control, cancer pain.

Patients who undergo surgery, radiation therapy, or chemotherapy to reduce the cancer usually continue to take pain medications until the cancer treatment shows effects. Some patients may continue to take them if the cancer treatment is not completely effective in relieving their pain.

Palliative Radiation Therapy

Tumors often cause pain when they get large enough to press on surrounding nerves. Radiation therapy can be used to shrink such tumors, which can reduce pain. Often a single dose of radiation therapy is all that is needed to relieve pain. Doctors also use radiation to relieve symptoms such as bleeding, difficulty swallowing, blockage of the intestines, compression of blood vessels or nerves by tumors, and potential fractures that could occur as a result of cancer that has spread, or metastasized, to bones.

Radiation treatment sometimes enhances the effectiveness of analgesic medicines and other noninvasive therapies because it directly targets the cancer causing the pain. Treatment is supervised by a radiation oncologist, a doctor who specializes in the use of radiation for cancer patients.

The success of radiation to relieve symptoms depends on factors such as the type and location of the cancer, as well as the radiation energy source, dose of radiation, and length of treatment. Several methods of radiation therapy are available.

External Beam Radiation

External beam radiation uses a radiotherapy machine that emits high-energy rays capable of killing cancer cells. The radiation oncologist calculates the dose of radiation needed to kill cancer cells while causing the fewest side effects, and then focuses the beam of radiation on cancer cells, even when they are deep inside the body. External beam radiation may involve multiple treatments over several days or weeks.

Internal Radiation (Brachytherapy)

Another method of delivering radiation involves placing small pellets or metal rods containing radioactive materials into or next to a tumor. Each pellet is about the size of a grain of rice and is placed so that the small amount of radiation each one produces can do the most damage to cancer cells while sparing healthy surrounding tissue. The pellets are usually implanted during a simple surgical procedure. This method is called internal radiation, interstitial radiation, or brachytherapy. Sometimes both internal and external beam radiation therapies are used together for palliative purposes.

Radiopharmaceuticals

A radiopharmaceutical is a medicine that contains a radioactive substance. It is injected into a vein to travel to areas where cancer has spread. The radiation emitted by the drug kills cancer cells, thereby relieving pain. This type of radiotherapy is used primarily to treat patients whose pain results from bone metastases. For patients whose cancer has spread to many bones, injection of radioactive medicines is far more effective than aiming external beam radiation at each affected bone.

Sometimes a single injection can bring extensive pain relief within a week, and the effects often last for several months. This procedure can be repeated if bone pain returns. In some cases, radiopharmaceuticals are used together with external beam radiation aimed at the most painful bone metastases. This approach has helped many men with prostate cancer, but its usefulness against other cancers is not as well documented. Examples of radiopharmaceuticals include strontium-89, iodine-131, rhenium-186, and samarium-153.

Side Effects of Radiation Therapy

Dose levels of radiation used for palliative treatment are lower than those used for primary treatment of cancers, so side effects are generally mild. Still, patients may experience a variety of undesirable reactions to radiation therapy.

External beam radiation may cause skin to redden or tan. Both effects gradually fade. If the neck area is treated with external beam radiation, the thyroid gland may be damaged, requiring the patient to take thyroid hormone replacement pills. Radiation directed to the head and neck may damage the salivary glands, resulting in dry mouth, sore throat, hoarseness, difficulty swallowing, partial or complete loss of taste, and temporary fatigue. Radiation of the abdomen can lead to nausea, diarrhea, vomiting, and temporary or permanent damage to the intestines. Chest radiation may cause lung scarring that can lead to shortness of breath. Radiation therapy directed at the brain may cause subtle problems with thinking, but the extent depends on the dose used and may not occur until years after treatment.

While radiopharmaceuticals initially travel throughout the body after injection, potential side effects are basically limited to a few areas. Some patients experience a "flare" or increase in bone pain several days after the injection, which subsides after a few days. Because these drugs tend to concentrate in the bones, the bone marrow may be affected, which can lead to anemia and to an increased risk of bleeding or infection. These drugs are removed from the body through the urine, so some patients may develop cystitis (inflammation of the bladder).

Will I Become Radioactive?

You will not become permanently radioactive if you undergo radiation therapy. External radiation therapy affects targeted cells only for a moment. With internal radiation therapy, your body may or may not emit a small amount of radiation for a short time. Precautions are taken anyway and may include hospitalization and limitation of visitors. (Pregnant women—whose fetuses are vulnerable to the smallest doses of radiation—and children are not allowed to visit.) Patients who are given radioactive substances such as iodine, phosphorus, or strontium by mouth or into a vein are kept isolated until their bodies no longer contain enough radioactivity to be hazardous to others. Be sure to discuss any safety concerns you have and precautions you should take with your radiation oncologist, nurse, or the radiation safety officer at your treatment facility.

How Radiation Therapy Is Used to Control or Relieve Symptoms

Radiation therapy may be used to:

- relieve bone pain, especially that caused by metastasis from breast, lung, or prostate cancer
- relieve pain caused by tumors pressing on or invading nerves
- control bleeding caused by tumors
- reduce pain caused by tumors that ulcerate, such as certain breast cancers, head and neck cancers, and skin cancers
- ease breathing problems (dyspnea), coughing, or chest pains caused by tumors that block the breathing passages
- reduce pain caused by large abdominal tumors
- relieve pain from tumors that press on the spinal cord or that cause back pain, leg weakness, shooting pains, sphincter problems, or numbness
- relieve headaches caused by inoperable brain tumors that press on the skull
- shrink tumors blocking hollow organs or tubes, such as the bronchial tubes, esophagus, bile ducts, ureters, lymph channels, blood vessels, gynecologic system, or gastrointestinal tracts
- relieve problems caused when the tumors grow in small, constricted spaces

While Bruce's condition was not curable, his doctor explained to him that chemotherapy might shrink the cancer and relieve some of his symptoms. After two cycles of chemotherapy with gemcitabine (Gemzar), he needed less medication each day to control his pain, and the whites of his eyes returned to normal. A CT scan showed that the cancerous tumors were now about half their original size. He underwent two more cycles of chemotherapy, after which the tumors appeared to remain the same size. The cancer was no longer shrinking, and his doctor decided to give him a break from the chemotherapy, because he had been experiencing severe diarrhea.

Palliative Chemotherapy

While surgery and radiation therapy are generally used to treat localized cancers, chemotherapy is used to treat cancer that has spread to other parts of the body. Depending on the type of cancer and its stage (extent of spread in the body), chemotherapy can be used to cure cancer, to keep the cancer from spreading, to slow the cancer's growth, or to kill cancer cells that may have spread to other parts of the body. Chemotherapy drugs may also be used to relieve pain caused by growing tumors or to relieve other symptoms caused by cancer. Chemotherapy is used to reduce the size of a tumor causing pain. It is not effective for all patients, and pain relief with this method is usually slow, if it occurs at all.

The drugs used in chemotherapy are most often given by injection into a vein or by mouth (in pill form). They enter the bloodstream and travel to all areas of the body. Often a combination of chemotherapy drugs is used.

Side Effects of Chemotherapy

Side effects of chemotherapy depend on the type of drugs used, the amount taken, and the length of treatment. Some of the most common side effects are nausea and vomiting, fatigue, temporary hair loss, mouth sores, and increased chance of bleeding and infections. Chemotherapy side effects can also lead to other types of pain. Some side effects may be harder to cope with, while others may be mild. Most side effects can be controlled with medications, supportive care measures, or by changing the treatment schedule.

Hormonal Therapy

Hormones are chemical messengers that regulate many functions in different parts of the body. Some types of cancer, especially breast, prostate, and endometrial cancer, grow in response to hormones normally circulating in the blood. In these types of cancer, drugs can be given to lower certain hormone levels, which can slow or stop tumor growth. Sometimes different hormones must be combined before cancer responds, and results might take several weeks to become apparent. Hormonal therapy does not cure cancer. However, the treatment is capable of providing enduring cancer pain relief without causing some of the more serious side effects seen with chemotherapy. Because hormonal therapy lowers the levels of the major male or female hormones, side effects are often related to sexual function (such as impotence in men and vaginal dryness in women). Hot flashes are also common.

Bisphosphonate Therapy

Bisphosphonates are a group of drugs that slow down the action of bone cells called osteoclasts. Osteoclasts are cells that normally eat away small pieces of bone, allowing other cells to reform the proper shape of the bone. When cancer spreads to the bones, osteoclasts may become overactive, which can lead to bone pain. Bisphosphonates are used to treat pain in the bones from multiple myeloma as well as from breast or prostate cancer. They are usually given in cycles similar to those used for chemotherapy, although their side effects are less severe.

Three months after the completion of his chemotherapy, Bruce began to notice the yellow returning to his eyes and in the skin of his face as well. The abdominal pain was again difficult to control with pain medication. A CT scan showed that his pancreas had grown again and was preventing the liver from emptying its bile into the intestines, which was causing his jaundice. After consulting with his doctor, Bruce underwent a stent placement, a surgical procedure to relieve the obstruction of the flow of bile. Within a week, his skin returned to normal and his pain was successfully relieved with lower doses of medicine.

Palliative Surgery

Surgery is generally considered when there is a good chance that it will improve a person's quality of life by reducing pain or decreasing the need for high doses of medication that cause unpleasant side effects. Surgery may involve reducing the size of, or debulking, a tumor that presses on nerves, or removing organs that aggravate cancer symptoms. While results vary depending on the type and size of the tumor and the procedure being performed, in some cases surgery may lead to longer-term symptom-free survival.

Surgery may also be performed to prevent further damage to the patient's body. For example, cancer that has spread to bones can weaken them, leading to fractures (breaks) that tend to heal very poorly. An operation to reinforce a bone with a metal rod can prevent some fractures and,

Surgery may be used to:
- unblock the intestines, bile ducts, or urinary system
- drain fluid that has built up in the abdomen
- gain access to an artery for injection of chemotherapy drugs
- remove or reduce the size of a pain-causing tumor that is unresponsive to other treatments

if the bone is already broken, can rapidly relieve pain and help the patient return to routine activities. Surgical treatment of metastatic cancer near the spinal cord or large nerves can prevent or relieve symptoms such as paralysis and severe pain.

Nerve Blocks

Over the next several months, Bruce's pain became more intense, until his medication was again no longer adequate. A temporary nerve block to his celiac plexus (a group of nerves in the abdomen) provided good relief but lasted only a few weeks. Knowing that this technique had worked before, his doctor recommended a permanent block of his celiac plexus to relieve his abdominal pain. Although he experienced some temporary diarrhea, the nerve block provided Bruce with pain relief for months.

There are hundreds of nerves in the body that can be compressed by tumors. Compression can cause pain in the areas of the body that a nerve goes through. This pain can be treated with a temporary or permanent nerve block, a procedure in which medicines, sometimes combined with other chemicals, are injected into or around nerves, disrupting their ability to transmit pain signals. Depending on the location, extent, and severity of pain, nerve blocks may be directed at individual nerves, nerve bundles and nerve roots, or into the spaces that enclose the spinal cord.

One way to think about a nerve block is by comparing it to cutting an electrical wire to interrupt the flow of electricity. Pain in the chest or abdominal wall can be relieved by interrupting nerve signals that travel from these sites up through the spinal cord. A similar nerve blocking process can be performed to treat any of hundreds of nerves in the body. Pain in the legs, groin, and lower back can be relieved by injecting medicines into the epidural space surrounding the spinal column or directly into the intrathecal space where the spinal cord itself is located.

Nerve blocks can be performed on an outpatient basis or during surgery. There is no way to predict exactly how effective a nerve block will be; the amount of pain relief depends on the location of the pain, the type of medications used, and the individual patient's response. Most people will experience at least some pain reduction from nerve blocks. However, patients with some types of pain may not benefit. Medical team members can perform both temporary and more permanent nerve blocks.

Temporary Nerve Blocks

Temporary nerve blocks involve the injection of local anesthetics, such as lidocaine or bupivicaine, into or near nerves. Many people routinely undergo temporary nerve blocks when they receive a shot of novocaine at the dentist's office. Another commonly used temporary nerve block is epidural anesthesia during childbirth.

Pain relief from a temporary nerve block often occurs immediately, but may last only a few hours and may need to be repeated frequently. Multiple injections may break a cycle of pain and inflammation, improve range of motion, and increase local blood flow. Doctors can repeat temporary nerve block injections as often as necessary because the procedure does not damage nerves. The addition of corticosteroid medicines (see chapter 5) often extends the duration of pain relief to days or even weeks. Corticosteroids reduce swelling, irritation, and inflammation that occur when tumors press on nerves. Nerve blocks are used not only to relieve pain caused directly by cancer, but also to relieve secondary pain, such as pain from muscle spasms, shingles, or nerve irritation.

Often, groups of nerves must be blocked simultaneously in order to achieve adequate pain relief. This may result in side effects in the area being treated such as muscle weakness or tingling and burning sensations. Nerve blocks may also cause loss of sensation and even temporary paralysis in affected areas. If the area includes certain nerve groups in the abdomen, low blood pressure or temporary loss of bladder or bowel control may result.

Permanent Nerve Blocks

When temporary nerve blocks do not relieve pain or must be constantly repeated, a permanent nerve block may be performed. Permanent nerve blocks involve the injection of chemicals that destroy portions of a nerve, thus blocking pain signals for long periods of time, often many months. These blocks are not always truly "permanent" because many peripheral nerve cells (those outside of the brain or spinal cord) have the ability to regenerate over time.

Permanent nerve blocks are also called destructive blocks, neurolytic blockades, or neuroablation. They are usually reserved for patients who do not respond well to temporary nerve blocks or for patients whose cancer is not expected to get better. The best candidates for permanent nerve blocks are patients whose source of pain is easily identified and not widespread. Doctors usually prefer to avoid administering permanent nerve blocks when pain covers a wide area (an exception is abdominal pain) or is located in different parts of the body that are not close to one another.

The chemicals used to kill nerve cells include ethanol and phenol, and are called neurolytic agents, or simply neurolytics. An injection of ethanol can be extremely painful for a short time and must be accompanied by a local anesthetic. Phenol has anesthetic properties of its own and causes no pain when injected.

Permanent nerve blocks require the skill of doctors who specialize in anesthesiology. Destroying precisely the right nerves or nerve bundles that are responsible for the pain requires a great deal of skill. Neurolytic chemicals kill nerves indiscriminately, harming any with which they come into contact. For that reason, a prognostic temporary nerve block is usually done first to determine precisely where to inject nerve-destroying chemicals. Even after a permanent nerve block is done, opioids at lower doses are often prescribed to help control any remaining pain.

Though the most commonly used method to kill nerves is to inject them with neurolytics, other options are available. During radiofrequency ablation, a special probe is heated to very high temperatures and then applied to nerve cells. Cryoanalgesia is another option, which involves the use of an extremely cold probe that freezes and kills nerves.

Side Effects of Nerve Blocks

Side effects of temporary nerve blocks are usually limited and typically include muscle weakness and loss of sensation, both of which wear off as the medicines are flushed from the body. But the side effects associated with permanent nerve blocks may be serious and irreversible and can include muscle weakness, numbness, paralysis, and incontinence, depending on which nerves are harmed by neurolytic chemicals. The closer nerve-killing agents are to the spinal cord, the more widespread side effects tend to be. Depending on where the nerves are located, the effects and side effects of nerve blocks differ.

Location of Nerve Blocks

Peripheral Nerve Blocks

Peripheral nerve blocks are most often used to treat pain in the head, chest, or abdomen. Peripheral nerves often overlap, requiring that more than one be blocked to relieve pain. These nerves transmit not only pain signals, but also information necessary for sensation and movement. When anesthetics are injected into peripheral nerves, they may interfere with these other activities and cause side effects, such as numbness or limited range of motion. Because of their potential for causing more serious side effects, peripheral nerve block procedures are performed very cautiously and should be preceded by diagnostic nerve blocks to gauge the possible effects of more permanent options.

Central Nerve Blocks

Central nerve blocks involve injections of anesthetics or neurolytic agents into the epidural space that surrounds the spinal cord or directly into the intrathecal space that houses the spinal cord itself. Temporary nerve blocks of this sort are regularly performed in hospitals to relieve back and neck pain and for women in labor.

For some patients whose pain is hard to control, a permanent or semi-permanent catheter (drug delivery tube) can be inserted between the vertebrae (bones of the spine) and into the epidural or intrathecal spaces. Doctors, nurses, or other caregivers can inject anesthetics as needed, or the medicines can be delivered automatically by special pumps. Because chemicals are injected close to nerve roots, very small amounts of anesthetics or neurolytic agents can produce profound pain relief. Even opioids such as morphine can be injected directly into nerves in or around the spinal cord.

Central nerve blocks are usually performed by specially trained anesthesiologists. Permanent central nerve blocks are even more complicated and require the expertise of other specialists. The procedures are safest when performed in the mid-back and riskier with more chance of side effects when performed in the neck and lower back.

Permanent nerve blocks performed in and around the spine carry many potential risks, including partial or total paralysis, loss of sensation, incontinence, and, rarely, cardiac or respiratory depression.

Sympathetic Nerve Blocks

Sympathetic nerves connect the central nervous system to internal organs. Sympathetic nerve blocks can be used to relieve pain in patients with pancreatic cancer and those with other tumors that cause abdominal and back pain. They can also be used to treat pain in the arms or legs that is unresponsive to other therapies. These nerve blocks can lead to several side effects, such as temporary low blood pressure, diarrhea, urinary difficulties, and weakness in the lower extremities.

Spinal Opioid Infusion

For patients who require repeated temporary blocks or whose pain is difficult to control, an alternative to a permanent nerve block may be an infusion catheter implanted intraspinally, meaning into the area of the spinal cord. Catheter implantation is a relatively pain-free and quick procedure. The catheter allows doctors to give strong analgesics such as morphine and fentanyl directly to nerves that cause pain. Medicines can be introduced as needed through the catheter with a syringe or automatically by an external infusion pump. In rare cases, tiny infusion pumps are surgically implanted inside the body, usually in the abdomen. These devices hold anesthetic reservoirs that last up to two months before a refill is required, but they are very expensive.

Because analgesic medicines are injected so close to the nerves, only small amounts are needed to produce significant, though temporary, pain relief. For example, patients who take morphine by mouth may need 100 to 1,000 mg per dose, compared with one to ten mg when the drug flows through a spinal catheter. As with oral medications, patients may develop tolerance to intraspinal opioids and require higher doses to establish adequate pain control.

A home care nurse is usually needed to monitor treatment and teach patients and family members how to use and maintain infusion pumps and catheters. Unlike the effects of permanent nerve blocks, those of intraspinal opioid treatment are temporary and reversible.

Continuous opioid infusion is relatively safe and has few unwanted effects, but the technique is reserved for patients in whom oral medications do not provide enough relief or cause too many side effects. A potential complication is infection at the site of the catheter implant, which can become serious because it lies so close to the spine. Intraspinal opioids may also cause bladder incontinence.

Neurosurgery

Neurosurgery (nerve surgery) for pain control involves surgically cutting or destroying nerves that transmit pain signals. It is used when other methods of pain control, including drug therapy and chemical nerve blocks, fail to provide sufficient relief. Because of the complexity, risks, and high costs, neurosurgery is rarely performed to relieve pain. Neurosurgery must be performed by neurosurgeons, specialists at highly equipped treatment centers. Neurosurgery is very expensive. Only patients with clearly localized pain are likely to benefit.

Nerve surgery is irreversible and involves serious risks, including the temporary or permanent loss of feeling or motor control in some parts of the body, impaired reflexes, inability to distinguish temperature changes, and incontinence.

Cordotomy is the nerve surgery most frequently performed to relieve pain. During the operation, the surgeon cuts nerves in the spinal cord with a scalpel or destroys them with a very hot electrode. Cordotomies are used to relieve leg or hip pain on one side of the body. The technique is usually not helpful for patients with pain in the upper body. Nine out of ten people who undergo a cordotomy report significant pain relief, but the pain returns within a year for about half of the patients. Potential complications of the procedure include mild paralysis, loss of coordination, and, most seriously, breathing difficulties.

Other pain relieving nerve surgeries include rhizotomy, during which a surgeon cuts nerves coming out of the spinal cord, and neurectomy, which is used to treat nerves on the surface of the body. These surgeries are uncommon.

CHAPTER 7

Complementary Nondrug Treatments

W hile going through cancer treatment, Daniel was bombarded with suggestions from friends about other methods he should try. Although people were just trying to help, it was confusing. He had also read a lot about complementary treatments, from relaxation and visualization to exercise and massage. He discussed all of these options with his doctor, who was able to help him decide what might work best for him.

◦◦◦

YOU MAY CONSIDER USING NONDRUG OR COMPLEMENTARY treatments for pain relief along with medications, surgery, or other medical procedures. These therapies can be very useful in helping to reduce pain and manage side effects and can be effectively used as part of a comprehensive pain-management effort.

Complementary therapies may also help you cope with the emotional and psychological impact of pain on your quality of life and well-being, both of which can be severely impacted by pain. For example, dealing with chronic pain can sometimes lead to depression or anxiety, which can make existing pain feel worse and decrease your desire to participate in family or social activities. Your mind can have a strong positive or negative influence on the way you cope with pain. Because of this potentially powerful mind and body connection, it is important for physicians and patients to consider the mind as well as the body in treating pain and to consider the use of complementary techniques as part of a comprehensive effort to control pain.

What Are Complementary Nondrug Treatments?

The American Cancer Society defines complementary treatments as supportive methods that are used to complement, or add to, conventional treatments. Complementary methods such as massage therapy, yoga, and meditation are also referred to as nondrug or noninvasive treatments. These techniques rely heavily on the ability of the mind to influence responses to pain. *Complementary methods do not alter the growth or spread of cancer.*

Complementary methods should not be confused with alternative therapies, which are unproven treatments sometimes used *instead of* conventional therapy to attempt to prevent, lessen, or cure disease. Alternative therapies may be harmful in and of themselves or may be dangerous because they are used instead of conventional medicine and thereby delay treatments that are proven to be helpful.

How Complementary Nondrug Treatments Can Help Control Pain

Medicines for cancer pain are used to treat the sensation and perception of pain—that is, what you feel. Nondrug treatments are aimed at reducing the emotional components of pain as well as how you respond to pain. Many of these treatments can increase your sense of personal control, reduce feelings of helplessness, provide opportunities to become actively involved in your own care, reduce stress and anxiety, elevate your mood, and raise your pain threshold.

Techniques such as meditation or distraction are designed to target how the mind processes pain. These methods can help you learn how to

It's helpful to gather as much information as possible about any complementary nondrug method you're interested in. Seek information from reputable, credible sources on the potential benefits and risks of the treatment you are considering. (See the *Resources* section of this book for sources you may want to consult.)

Let your health care team know you are considering a complementary treatment and that you want to make sure it will not interfere with the treatment prescribed for you. Develop a list of questions, and bring it along with any literature you wish to discuss with your health care team. Ask your doctor and nurse to be supportive partners in your education and treatment process.

Here are some sample questions you may want to ask your health care team and licensed practitioner about any methods you are interested in pursuing for your pain:

- Are there any nondrug methods you recommend as a part of my cancer treatment in order to help me deal with pain or anxiety?
- What can I expect from this method or treatment?
- Is there any complementary method I should avoid?
- What kind of experience do you have with nondrug treatments?
- Does my hospital or medical facility offer this method? If not, where can I go to find out more about it?
- Is the technique covered by my insurance? If not, what are the costs?
- Is this method widely available for use within the health care community, or is it controlled, with limited access to its use?

Questions to ask a licensed practitioner:

- Are you licensed or trained in this method?
- How many years have you been practicing this method?
- Is this method difficult to master?
- Can I be taught this technique so that I can practice it at home on my own?
- Are there any risks involved?
- Are there any books, videos, or other resources available that you can recommend?

relax and focus your thoughts away from the pain you are feeling, which lessens the effects of pain on your body.

Skin stimulation, which includes the use of cold and heat, massage, and other elements, can be used to block pain sensations or alter blood flow in the parts of the body being stimulated.

Complementary techniques such as prayer and yoga may help reduce feelings of anxiety or depression, which can increase the intensity of cancer pain.

The psychological and physical benefits of complementary nondrug treatments can have a very positive effect on your quality of life and well-being. Many of these methods are also used during cancer treatment to help ease painful side effects or uncomfortable physical symptoms.

Access to Complementary Nondrug Treatments

The medical community's interest in therapies that tap into the connection between the mind and body and their effects on healing and pain reduction has grown in recent years. Although research is still being done in this area, some treatments have been shown to be useful for dealing with cancer pain in particular, as outlined in this chapter.

Many treatment centers recognize that therapies such as biofeedback, music therapy, and counseling can help people with cancer deal with pain and its impact on their quality of life. Some centers have begun to offer these therapies as part of a comprehensive cancer treatment program. Many complementary methods are also taught or administered by health professionals, such as occupational and physical therapists, psychologists, social workers, or by other licensed and trained practitioners such as massage therapists, acupuncturists, members of the clergy, or music therapists.

Some mind and body techniques, such as yoga and relaxation, can be self-taught. Information is available through books, videos, and web sites. You may also find a class on some of these methods at fitness and community centers in your area, and some organizations can provide you with lists of licensed practitioners. The *Resources* section in the back of this book contains contact information for some helpful organizations.

Complementary techniques should be incorporated only as part of a comprehensive medical treatment plan that strives to help you cope both mentally and physically with your cancer pain. These methods can be safely used along with conventional treatment to help relieve symptoms or side effects, to ease pain, and to improve your quality of life.

Talk to members of your health care team about any nondrug treatments you are considering.

Complementary Nondrug Methods

The following techniques include methods that focus on the connections between the mind, body, and spirit and their power for healing, as well as methods that involve touching, manipulation, or movement of the body. When used along with conventional treatment, many of these methods can help relieve pain or improve your quality of life.

Acupuncture

According to a National Institutes of Health (NIH) expert panel consisting of scientists, researchers, and health care providers, acupuncture is an effective treatment for post-operative pain (as well as for nausea caused by chemotherapy drugs). Some evidence suggests that acupuncture may lessen the need for conventional pain-relief medicines. However, the NIH has not specifically recommended using acupuncture for cancer pain.

Acupuncture is a technique in which very thin needles of varying lengths are inserted through the skin. In traditional acupuncture, specially trained practitioners insert needles at specific locations, called acupoints, which are believed to control specific areas of pain sensation. Needles usually remain in place for less than 30 minutes. Skilled acupuncturists cause virtually no pain. Once inserted, the acupuncturist may twirl the needles and apply heat or

---

Insurance Coverage of Complementary Therapies

Many insurance companies are beginning to offer coverage of some of the more widely accepted complementary methods of treatment. In the year 2000, 30 major insurers, including Blue Cross and Medicare, covered at least one complementary method of treatment. Acupuncture is one of the complementary therapies most often covered by insurance companies. Contact your insurance company to find out what, if any, complementary services are covered by your plan.

If possible, you may wish to obtain a recommendation or referral from your doctor for the complementary therapy you are considering. Many insurance companies require that the method be shown to be reasonable and medically necessary, and it may help later on to have your doctor's recommendation. Insurance companies usually will not cover methods that have not been proven to be effective.

a weak electrical current to enhance the effects of therapy. In acupressure, a popular variation of acupuncture, therapists press on acupoints with their fingers instead of using needles. This technique is used by itself or as part of a larger system of manual healing such as shiatsu massage.

Although it originated 2,000 to 3,000 years ago, acupuncture remains an important component of current traditional Chinese medicine. In China, acupuncture is used as an anesthetic during surgery and is believed to have the power to cure diseases and relieve symptoms of illness. Some practitioners claim that acupuncture relieves pain by stimulating the production of endorphins—natural substances in the body responsible for relieving pain. In the United States and Europe, it is used primarily to control pain and relieve disease symptoms such as nausea.

Most doctors believe acupuncture is safe as long as the needles used are sterile and the therapy is conducted by a trained professional. The American Academy of Medical Acupuncture (323-937-5514; http://www.medicalacupuncture.org) maintains a current referral list of doctors who practice acupuncture. Medicare does not cover acupuncture, but it is covered by some private health insurance plans and health maintenance organizations.

Biofeedback

Biofeedback is a treatment method that uses monitoring devices to help people consciously regulate physiological (bodily) processes that are usually controlled automatically, such as heart rate, blood pressure, temperature, perspiration, and muscle tension.

Biofeedback has been approved by an independent panel convened by the NIH as a useful complementary therapy for treating chronic pain and insomnia. Biofeedback can also be used to regulate or alter other physical functions that may be causing discomfort. If you have chronic cancer-related pain, you might use biofeedback along with pain-relief medicines.

By learning to control heart rate, skin temperature, breathing rate, muscle control, and other physiological activity in the body, you can use biofeedback to reduce stress and muscle tension. Through a greater awareness of bodily functions, you can regulate or alter other physical functions that may cause discomfort. Perhaps the greatest benefit of biofeedback you may experience is the ability to reduce tension and promote relaxation, both of which can help you cope with your cancer pain.

With the help of special monitoring devices that provide feedback, you can learn to control certain body functions. A biofeedback therapist uses these monitoring devices to measure information that controls body processes and send messages to you indicating when the desired results are occurring. The process is repeated as often as necessary until you can reliably use conscious thought to change physical functions.

There are several different ways to measure body functions for biofeedback:

- Electromyogram (EMG) measures muscle tension. It is used to help heal muscle injuries and relieve chronic pain.
- Thermal biofeedback provides information about skin temperature, which is a good indicator of blood flow. Several health problems are related to blood flow, such as migraine headaches, anxiety, and high blood pressure.
- Electrodermal activity (EDA) shows changes in perspiration rates. It is used in treating anxiety.
- Finger pulse measurements are used to reflect high blood pressure, heartbeat irregularities, and anxiety.
- Breathing rate is monitored to promote relaxation.

Biofeedback requires a trained and certified professional to control monitoring equipment and interpret changes. Check with your medical facility to see if they offer biofeedback therapy.

Distraction

Distraction is a technique used to turn your attention to something other than what you may be feeling. When used along with effective pain medicines, distraction can help decrease anxiety, pain, fatigue, and muscle tension. It can also increase your confidence in your ability to handle pain. Because this technique does not require much energy, it may be useful when you tired. Slow, rhythmic breathing can also be used for distraction as well as for relaxation.

Many people use this method without realizing it when they watch television or listen to the radio to "take their minds off" the pain. Some people find it helpful to listen to fast music through a headset or earphones. When listening to music, you may find it helpful adjust the volume to match the intensity of pain, making it louder when you feel very severe pain. To help keep your attention on the music, you can tap out the rhythm.

Any activity that occupies your attention can be used for distraction. For example, losing yourself in a good book or going to a movie might divert your mind from pain. If you find it difficult to concentrate, you may try math games, like subtracting 123 from 1,000, or counting back from a certain number. If you enjoy working with your hands, crafts such as needlework, model building, or painting may distract you from pain.

If you are tired, irritable, and feel more pain after using a distraction technique, or if you are experiencing severe pain, you may want to use distraction carefully or privately. You can find out more about this technique by asking someone on your health care team or by contacting the American Cancer Society (800-ACS-2345; http://www.cancer.org).

Exercise

Exercise is the performance of physical activity that requires energy expenditure. It is important to exercise regularly to keep muscles functioning as well as possible. Regular exercise can help increase your energy level, reduce pain, and contribute to your well-being. Exercise can also prevent problems associated with immobility, such as stiff joints, breathing problems, constipation, skin sores, poor appetite, and mental changes.

Aerobic exercise (such as walking, jogging, cycling, yoga, and swimming) increases blood flow to the heart and increases the oxygen going into the lungs. Regular aerobic exercise can also lower blood cholesterol, strengthen bones, raise metabolism, and increase endurance. Anaerobic exercise (such as strength training) is essential for developing muscles, strength, speed, and power, and for maintaining freedom of movement. An ideal exercise program should combine aerobic and anaerobic exercises.

The American Cancer Society recommends 30 minutes or more of regular exercise several times a week. The 30 minutes does not need to be continuous to be beneficial. You can accomplish this goal of 30 minutes by walking briskly (three to four miles per hour) for about two miles or through a variety of other activities, including jogging, swimming, gardening, housework, or dancing at a level of intensity equivalent to brisk walking. It's important when exercising to try to maintain a positive attitude, set reasonable goals, and stick to a regular exercise program.

Some form of physical activity is beneficial to everyone, even someone confined to a bed. Most people can perform range-of-motion exercises and general stretching. In fact, pain medication combined with stretching exercises is one of the best solutions for keeping comfortable when confined to bed. Inactivity can lead to muscle weakness, pain in joints or legs, and other problems such as poor or no appetite, constipation, skin sores, problems with breathing, and mental changes. Performing range-of-motion exercises as instructed by your nurse, doctor, or physical therapist can help alleviate some of these problems.

Exercise can provide benefits to your mind as well as your body. Physical activities may improve your sense of being in touch with your body. Regular exercise can also induce feelings of relaxation and optimism and may help decrease feelings of inadequacy and helplessness. For many people, exercise provides a sense of accomplishment and control, which is especially helpful to people who may be feeling depressed. Exercise also has a calming affect on many people and can be a form of distraction from pain.

Before you begin an exercise program, talk with your doctor, who will take into account your particular circumstances so that a program of exercise can be tailored to your situation. This will allow you to learn the best types of exercise for maintaining your health, the level of activity appropriate for you, and signs to watch for that might indicate over-exertion. Pushing yourself too hard may be discouraging and could result in injury. Be aware that some treatments limit physical activity. Be sure to ask about activities you should avoid.

Your doctor should be able to recommend an exercise professional or physical therapist to help you get started. You can also check with the YWCA (800-YWCA-US1; http://www.ywca.org), YMCA (888-333-YMCA; http://www.ymca.net), or American Heart Association (800-AHA-USA1; http://www.americanheart.org) for information on exercise programs.

Humor Therapy

Humor therapy is the use of humor for the relief of physical and emotional difficulties. It is used as a technique to promote health and cope with illness. Laughter can stimulate the circulatory system by increasing heart rate and oxygen use. The use of humor can sometimes lead to an increase in pain tolerance.

For many people, humor therapy can provide a welcome distraction from pain. It is useful for treating people with physical and emotional problems. It is generally used to provide some pain relief, encourage relaxation, and reduce stress. Being able to find humor in everyday events is thought to be helpful. As with so many mind and body connections, humor seems to provide temporary relief from worry and can lead to an overall sense of well-being. Physically, laughter exercises the same muscles and organs we use for breathing, promoting relaxation and reducing stress.

Many hospitals and ambulatory care centers have incorporated special rooms where materials—and sometimes people—are used to help make people laugh. Materials include movies, audio and videotapes, books, games, and puzzles for patients of every age. Many hospitals also use volunteer groups who visit patients for the purpose of providing opportunities for laughter.

Hypnosis

Hypnosis is one of several relaxation methods that have been approved by an independent panel, convened by the NIH, as a useful complementary therapy for treating chronic pain. People with cancer can use hypnosis to reduce pain, promote relaxation, and reduce stress. Hypnosis can also lower blood pressure and anxiety and can be used to reduce nausea, vomiting, phobias, and aversions to certain cancer treatments. People who are hypnotized have selective attention and are able to achieve a state of heightened concentration while blocking out distractions. Under hypnosis, people can achieve a state of restful alertness that helps them focus on a certain problem or symptom. This allows them to be open to images, suggestions, and ideas for resolving issues and improving their quality of life.

There are many different types of hypnotic techniques; however, most hypnosis begins with an induction. While a person is sitting or lying quietly, the hypnotherapist talks in gentle, soothing tones, describes images, and repeats a series of verbal suggestions that allow you to become relaxed, yet deeply absorbed and focused on your awareness. People under hypnosis may appear to be asleep, but they are actually in an altered state of concentration and can focus on a specific goal. During hypnosis, a person is very receptive to suggestions made by the hypnotherapist. To relieve pain, the therapist may suggest that pain will be gone when the person "wakes up." Some cancer patients have learned methods of self-hypnosis that they use to control pain.

Contrary to what many believe, people under hypnosis are not under the control of the hypnotherapist, nor can they be made to do something they do not want to do. Hypnosis will not work if the person does not want to be hypnotized. Hypnosis is not brainwashing and ideas are not "planted" in people's minds to make people do things against their will. Quite the opposite is true. Hypnosis is used to help people gain more control over their actions, emotions, and bodies. People may relieve pain through intense concentration to block their natural responses to pain.

Health care professionals, including physicians, psychotherapists, and social workers, can perform hypnosis. People who practice hypnosis are licensed. It is important to be hypnotized by a trained professional. Ask your doctor for more information about where to find a qualified hypnotherapist, or contact the American Society for Clinical Hypnosis (630-980-4740; http://www.asch.net).

Imagery and Visualization

Imagery involves the use of mental exercises and relaxation techniques designed to enable the mind to influence the health and well-being of the body. It is like a deliberate daydream that actively involves all of the senses. Imagery is considered to be similar to meditation (see page 131). Some people have found that imagery can relieve physical pain and emotional anxiety, improve the effectiveness of drug therapies, and provide emotional insights. Imagery is also used in biofeedback and hypnosis.

Imagery Exercise for Pain

Ball of Energy

The following is an exercise using the image of a ball of energy:

1. Close your eyes. Breathe slowly and feel yourself relax.
2. Concentrate on your breathing. Breathe slowly and comfortably from your abdomen. Breathe in this slow rhythm for a few minutes.
3. Imagine a ball of healing energy forming in your lungs or on your chest. It may be like a white light. It can be vague. It does not have to be vivid.
4. Imagine this ball forming, taking shape. Sometimes imagining pouring cool water on a burning pain or sensation is useful.
5. When you are ready, imagine that the air you breathe in blows this healing ball of energy to the area of your pain. Once there, the ball heals and relaxes you.
6. When you breathe out, imagine the air blows the ball away from your body. As it goes, the ball takes your pain with it. (Do not blow as you breathe out. Breathe out naturally.)
7. Repeat the last two steps each time you breathe in and out.
8. You may imagine that the ball gets bigger and bigger as it takes more and more discomfort away from your body.
9. To end the imagery, count slowly to three, breathe in deeply, open your eyes, and say silently to yourself, "I feel alert and relaxed."
10. Begin moving about slowly.

credited to Dr. David E. Bresler, President, Academy for Guided Imagery, Malibu, CA.

Some people with cancer use imagery to reduce the nausea and vomiting associated with chemotherapy, relieve stress, enhance the immune system, promote weight gain, or fight depression. It is also thought that focusing on certain images may reduce pain both during imagery and for hours afterward, although how this works is not completely understood.

There are a variety of imagery techniques. One common technique, guided imagery, involves visualizing a specific image or goal to be achieved and then imagining achieving that goal. Guided imagery can be helpful in managing stress, anxiety, and depression, and in lowering blood pressure, pain, and the side effects of chemotherapy. It can also be valuable in easing anxiety related to radiation therapy, including fears about the equipment, surgical pain, and recurrence of cancer. Imagery for pain relief is usually done with the eyes closed. A relaxation technique may be used first. The image can be something such as a ball of healing energy or a picture drawn in your mind of yourself as a person without pain.

Imagery techniques can be learned with the help of books and tapes, or they can be practiced under the guidance of a trained therapist. Imagery sessions with a health professional may last 20 to 30 minutes. Ask your nurse or doctor if information about imagery techniques is available at your medical facility.

Meditation

Meditation is a mind-body method that uses concentration or reflection to relax the body and calm the mind in order to create a sense of well-being. To meditate is to ponder, to think about, or to reflect upon. The ultimate goal of meditation is to separate oneself mentally from the outside world. The NIH National Center for Complementary and Alternative Medicine reports that regular meditation can increase longevity and the quality of life and reduce chronic pain, anxiety, high blood pressure, and blood cortisol levels initially brought on by stress.

Meditation can be a helpful relaxation method when used as a complementary method for treating chronic pain and some of the side effects of pain, including insomnia, stress, and anxiety. Successful meditation can result in clearing the mind of all distractions, including those that create stress, discomfort, worry, and fear, all of which can increase the sensation of pain for people with cancer.

According to practitioners, meditation should be performed once or twice a day for 15 to 20 minutes. A quiet room where a person can sit comfortably is needed. Typically, a meditator will sit with closed eyes and attempt to achieve a feeling of peace until a relaxed yet alert state is reached. To reach this state, a person will concentrate on a pleasant idea or thought, chant a phrase or special sound (sometimes called a mantra), or focus on the sound of his or her own breathing. Although meditation is usually done while sitting, there are some forms which involve movement like tai chi, aikido (a Japanese martial art), and walking (such as in Zen Buddhism).

Meditation can be performed without an instructor or it can be guided by yoga masters, doctors, or mental health professionals such as psychiatrists. Some clinics at major medical centers and local hospitals practice meditation as a form of behavioral medicine. Information about meditation can also be found in books and videotapes.

Music Therapy

Music therapy is a method that consists of the active or passive use of music in order to promote healing and enhance the quality of life. There is some evidence that when used along with conventional medical treatment, music therapy can help to reduce pain and anxiety (as well as relieve chemotherapy-induced nausea and vomiting). It may also relieve stress and provide an overall sense of well-being, which can be important factors for a person living with chronic pain. Some medical experts believe music can aid healing and improve physical movement. Music therapy may also reduce high blood pressure, rapid heartbeat, breathing rate, depression, and sleeplessness.

Some aspects of music therapy include music improvisation, receptive music listening, songwriting, lyric discussion, imagery, music performance, and learning through music. Individuals can also perform their own music therapy by listening to music or sounds at home.

Music therapists design sessions for individuals and groups based on individual needs and tastes. Music therapy can be conducted in a variety of places, including hospitals, cancer centers, hospices, at home, or anywhere people can benefit from its calming or stimulating effects.

There are currently over 5,000 professional music therapists working in health care settings in the United States today. They serve as part of cancer-management teams in many hospitals and cancer centers, helping to plan and evaluate treatment. Check with the American Music Therapy Association for more information (301-589-3300; http://www.namt.com).

Psychotherapy/Counseling

Psychotherapy, also referred to as counseling, covers a wide range of approaches designed to help people change their ways of thinking, feeling, or behaving. It may improve a person's quality of life by helping to reduce anxiety and depression, both of which can accompany pain and affect a person's sense of well-being. Therapy can also be beneficial for family members of people with cancer to help them deal with such feelings as anxiety or helplessness.

Psychotherapy can help you develop more effective coping strategies for dealing with cancer and some of its side effects, such as pain and stress. It can also teach you ways to communicate better with your doctor and allow you to more closely follow medical instructions because you feel your own needs are being recognized. Therapy may be conducted individually, as well as in couples, families, and groups (see chapter 2 for more information).

Relaxation

Relaxation exercises are used to relieve some types of pain or to keep it from getting worse by reducing tension in the muscles. They can increase energy, reduce fatigue and anxiety, promote sleep, and make other pain-relief methods work better. For example, some people find that relaxation techniques enhance the effectiveness of pain medication.

There are a number of different relaxation methods, a few of which are listed here:

- **Visual concentration** involves opening your eyes and staring at an object or closing your eyes and thinking of a peaceful, calm scene.
- **Rhythmic massage** is done with the palm of your hand by firmly massaging an area of pain in a circular motion.
- **Inhaling and exhaling** involve breathing in deeply while tensing your muscles or a group of muscles, holding your breath and keeping muscles tense for a second or two, and then letting go and breathing out while letting your body go limp.
- **Slow rhythmic breathing** can be practiced by staring at an object or by closing your eyes and concentrating on your breathing or on a peaceful scene.
- **Progressive muscle relaxation** involves learning how to relax different muscle groups throughout your body.

Relaxation Exercises You Can Try

Visual concentration and rhythmic massage:
- Open your eyes and stare at an object, or close your eyes and think of a peaceful, calm scene.
- With the palm of your hand, massage near the area of pain in a firm, circular motion. Avoid red, raw, swollen, or tender areas. You may wish to ask a family member or friend to do this for you.

Inhale/tense, exhale/relax:
- Inhale (breathe in) deeply. At the same time, tense your muscles or a group of muscles. For example, you can squeeze your eyes shut, frown, clench your teeth, make a fist, or stiffen your arms and legs as tightly as you can.
- Hold your breath and keep muscles tense for a second or two.
- Let go! Exhale and let your body go limp.

Slow rhythmic breathing:
- Stare at an object or close your eyes and concentrate on your breathing or on a peaceful scene.
- Take a slow, deep breath.
- As you breathe out, relax your muscles and feel the tension draining.
- Now remain relaxed and begin breathing slowly and comfortably, concentrating on your breathing. Just breathe naturally. If you ever feel out of breath, take a deep breath and then continue the slow breathing exercise.
- Each time you breathe out, concentrate on relaxing and going limp. If some muscles are not relaxed, such as your shoulders, focus on them and relax them as you breathe out. You need to do this only once or twice for each specific muscle group.
- Continue slow, rhythmic breathing for a few seconds up to ten minutes, depending on your need.
- To end your slow rhythmic breathing, count silently and slowly from one to three. Open your eyes. Say silently to yourself, "I feel alert and relaxed." Begin moving about slowly.

Other methods include using imagery (see *Imagery* on page 129) and listening to slow, familiar music through an earphone or headset.

Relaxation may be practiced sitting up or lying down. Choose a quiet place whenever possible. Close your eyes. Do not cross your arms and legs; that might cut off circulation and cause numbness or tingling. If you are lying down, be sure you are comfortable; relaxation will not work if it is forced. It may take up to two weeks of practice to feel the first results of relaxation. It should be practiced for at least five to ten minutes twice a day.

Relaxation may be difficult to use with severe pain. However, you may be able to use a simple relaxation method such as visual concentration with rhythmic massage or simply breathe in and tense your muscles, then breathe out and relax. Sometimes breathing too deeply for a while can cause shortness of breath. If this is a problem, take shallow breaths and/or breathe more slowly. If you experience a feeling of "suffocation," take a deep breath and exhale slowly, trying not to focus on your breathing. *Do not continue any relaxation technique that increases your pain, makes you feel uneasy, or causes any unpleasant effects.*

Various relaxation tapes are commercially available that can provide step-by-step instructions in relaxation techniques. If you have trouble using these methods, ask your doctor or nurse to refer you to a therapist who is experienced in relaxation techniques.

Skin Stimulation

Skin stimulation is the use of pressure, friction, temperature change, or chemical substances to excite the nerve endings in the skin. Scientists believe that the same nerve pathways transmit sensations of pain directly to the brain. When the skin is stimulated so that pressure, warmth, or cold is felt, pain sensation is lessened or blocked. Skin stimulation also alters the flow of blood to the affected area. Skin stimulation may lessen or eliminate pain during the stimulation and for hours after it is finished.

Stimulation is done either on or near the area of pain. You also can use skin stimulation on the side of the body opposite of the pain. For example, you might stimulate the left knee to decrease pain in the right knee. Stimulating the skin in areas away from the pain can be used to increase relaxation and may relieve pain.

Cold or Heat Applications
Cold applications are often used to reduce pain by numbing the affected area with gel packs or ice. Gel packs work well because they are soft and

flexible even when frozen and can be reused as often as necessary. (Gel packs are available at drugstores and medical supply stores.) An ice pack or ice cubes wrapped in a towel can also be effective.

Heat applications are generally used to soothe painful or sore muscles. A heating pad that generates its own moisture is useful for this purpose. Other heat applications include heated gel packs, hot water bottles, hot towels, a regular heating pad, or a hot bath or shower.

It is important to remember that heat and cold applications can easily damage skin. Extreme heat or cold can burn your skin. When using either method, you should limit your exposure to five to ten minutes and do not use any application over any area where your circulation or sensation is poor.

Massage

A growing number of health care professionals recognize massage as a useful addition to conventional medical treatment. Massage can relieve stress, anxiety, and pain. It involves manipulating, rubbing, and kneading the body's muscle and soft tissue. For pain relief, it is most effective when slow, steady, circular motions are used. Massage can be applied over or near the area of pain with bare hands or with any substance that feels good, such as talcum powder, warm oil, or hand lotion. Depending upon where your pain is located, you may massage yourself or ask a family member or friend to give you a massage. Having someone give you a foot rub, back rub, or hand rub can be very relaxing and may relieve pain. Some people find brushing or stroking lightly more comforting than deep massage. Use whatever works best for you.

There is a wide range of training and certification available for massage therapists. Not all states require licensing, but it may be helpful to use a massage therapist who has experience and training in helping clients who suffer from cancer pain.

Menthol

Many menthol preparations are available for pain relief. When they are rubbed into the skin, they increase blood circulation to the affected area and produce a warm (sometimes cool) soothing feeling that lasts for several hours. There are creams, lotions, liniments, or gels that contain menthol. Brands include Ben-Gay, Icy Hot, Mineral Ice, and Heat.

Some Warnings about the Use of Skin Stimulation

- If skin stimulation increases your pain, stop using it.
- Avoid massage and vibration over red, raw, tender, or swollen areas.
- If you are having radiation therapy, check with your doctor or nurse before using skin stimulation. Do not apply ointments, salves, or liniments to the treatment area, and do not use heat or extreme cold on treated areas. Avoid massage in the treated area.
- Many menthol preparations contain an ingredient similar to aspirin. A small amount of this aspirin-like substance is absorbed through the skin. If you have been told not to take aspirin, do not use these preparations until you check with your doctor.
- Do not rub menthol preparations over broken skin, a skin rash, or mucous membranes (such as inside your mouth or around your rectum). Make sure you do not get the menthol in your eyes.
- Do not use heat over a new injury because it can increase bleeding. Wait at least 24 hours.
- Never use a heating pad on bare skin or go to sleep with it turned on. Be careful while using a heating pad if you do not have much feeling in the area on which you are using it.
- Do not use cold so intense or for so long that the cold itself causes pain. If you start to shiver when using cold, stop using it right away.

Before using a menthol preparation over a large area, test a small amount of the preparation in a circle about one inch in diameter in the area of pain (or the area to be stimulated). This will let you know whether the menthol is uncomfortable to you or irritates your skin.

Pressure

Pressure can be applied with the entire hand or the base, the fingertip, knuckle, or the ball of the thumb. It is usually most effective when applied as firmly as possible without causing pain. You can use pressure for up to one minute. This often will relieve pain for several minutes to several hours after the pressure is released.

You may want to experiment by applying pressure for about ten seconds to various areas over or near your pain to see if it helps. You can also feel around your pain and outward to see if you can find "trigger points," small areas under the skin that are especially sensitive or that trigger pain.

Vibration

Vibration can also be used to bring temporary relief over or near an area of pain. For example, the scalp attachment of a hand-held vibrator often relieves a headache. For low back pain, a vibrator placed at the small of the back may be helpful. You may also use a vibrating device such as a small battery-operated vibrator, a handheld electric vibrator, a large heat-massage electric pad, a bed vibrator, or a vibrating chair. These devices can usually be found at your local drug store or medical supply store.

Some of the stimulation methods listed above may be helpful in reducing your pain. You may want to experiment with different methods to see which ones work best for you. If you are not sure which you should or should not try, talk to your nurse or doctor about your options.

Spirituality and Prayer

Spirituality is generally described as an awareness of something greater than the individual and is usually expressed through religion or prayer. Spirituality and religion are very important to the quality of life for some people with cancer. Intercessory prayer (praying for others) may be an effective addition to conventional medical care. The benefits of prayer may include the reduction of stress and anxiety, the promotion of a more positive outlook, and the strengthening of the will to live, all of which can have a significant impact on your life if you are coping with chronic pain.

People who practice various forms of spirituality claim that prayer can decrease the negative effects of disease (such as pain), speed recovery, and increase the effectiveness of medical treatments. Because the pain and side effects of cancer may be overwhelming, regular participation in spiritual practices such as prayer can help to provide better coping skills and enhance well-being for some people. Religious attendance has been associated with improvement of various health conditions such as cancer as well as improved overall health status.

There are many forms of spirituality. The most common involve prayer and regular attendance at religious ceremonies, usually at churches, synagogues, temples, or other houses of worship. Prayer, which can be performed alone or in a group, may be silent or spoken out loud and can take place in any setting. Spirituality in the form of religious attendance may also involve praying for oneself or for others. In this type of setting, the entire congregation may be asked to pray for a sick person or the person's family. Some religions set aside certain times of the day and special days of the week for prayer. Standard prayers written by religious leaders are often memorized and repeated during private sessions and in groups. Prayers often ask a higher being for help, understanding, wisdom, or strength in dealing with life's problems.

Many medical institutions and practitioners include spirituality and prayer as important components of healing. In addition, hospitals have chapels, and they contract with religious leaders and voluntary organizations to serve the spiritual needs of people with cancer. Information about local religious organizations in your area should be available in your local phone directory.

Transcutaneous Electrical Nerve Stimulation (TENS)

Transcutaneous electrical nerve stimulation (TENS) is a method of pain relief in which a special device transmits electrical impulses through electrodes to an area of the body that is in pain. Supporters claim that TENS is an effective method for relieving acute pain caused by surgery, migraines, injuries, arthritis, tendonitis, bursitis, chronic wounds, cancer, and other sources. Some people with cancer, particularly those with mild neuropathic pain (pain related to nerve tissue damage), may benefit from TENS for brief periods of time. TENS may also be more effective when used with pain medicines. Although there is some evidence that TENS may offer short-term pain relief for some people, the long-term benefits have not been proven.

A TENS system consists of an electrical generator connected by wires to a pair of electrodes. The electrodes are attached to the patient's skin near the source of pain. When the generator is switched on, a mild electrical current travels through the electrodes into the body. Patients may feel tingling or warmth during treatment. A session typically lasts from five to 15 minutes, and treatments may be applied as often as necessary, depending on the severity of pain.

TENS is used widely by physical therapists and other medical practitioners, but can also be performed at home by patients using a portable TENS system. There are more than 100 types of TENS units approved for use by the Food and Drug Administration. A prescription is needed to obtain a system, so if you are interested in obtaining a home TENS unit, you will need to talk to your doctor or physical therapist.

Yoga

Yoga is a form of nonaerobic exercise that involves a program of precise posture and breathing activities. Yoga is one of the oldest mind and body health systems in existence and was first practiced in India over 5,000 years ago. According to a report to the NIH, there is some evidence to suggest yoga may be useful as a complementary method to help relieve symptoms associated with cancer, high blood pressure, and other conditions. Research has also shown that yoga can be used to control physiological functions such as heart rate, respiration, metabolism, body temperature, brain waves, skin resistance, and other bodily functions.

People who practice yoga claim that it leads to a state of physical health, relaxation, happiness, peace, and tranquility. There is some evidence showing that yoga can lower stress, increase strength, and provide a good form of exercise. Proponents also claim that yoga can be used to eliminate insomnia and increase stamina. Yoga may help a person with cancer pain decrease stress and increase relaxation.

There are different variations and aspects of yoga. The most common form of yoga involves the use of movement, breathing exercises, and meditation to achieve a connection with the mind, body, and spirit. The goal of yoga is perfect concentration to attain the ancient Hindu ideal of samadhi—separation of pure consciousness from the outside world through the development of intuitive insight.

Practitioners claim yoga should be done either at the beginning or end of the day. A yoga session starts with the person sitting in an upright position and performing gentle movements, all of which are executed very slowly while taking slow, deep breaths from the abdomen. Yoga can be practiced at home without an instructor, in adult education classes, health clubs, and community centers. There are also numerous books and

- In order to avoid injury or increased pain, consult your doctor before beginning any exercise that may involve the manipulation of joints and muscles.
- Ask your doctor if he or she can recommend a certain complementary therapy that can help you with your particular kind of pain.
- Some insurance and health plans will cover at least some of the costs of several complementary techniques—such as acupuncture, biofeedback, and hypnosis—because these methods can be helpful in reducing pain and other side effects of treatment.
- Contact the National Institutes of Health National Center for Complementary and Alternative Medicine (NCCAM) for more information (888-644-6226; http://altmed.od.nih.gov).

videotapes available. A typical session can last between 20 minutes to one hour. A yoga session may include guided relaxation, meditation, and sometimes visualization. It often ends with the chanting of a mantra (a meaningful word or phrase) to achieve a deeper state of relaxation.

Some yoga postures are difficult to achieve. *Consult your doctor before beginning any exercise that may involve the manipulation of joints and muscles.*

CHAPTER 8

Managing Side Effects of Opioids

M *any people in pain believe the side effects of pain-relieving medications are worse than the pain itself. But Tom's pain was so severe that he was willing to accept the side effects in hopes of relieving his pain. He did experience constipation initially, but after his first episode, his anticonstipation treatment was regulated so that he had no more trouble with constipation. He was also sleepy, but when his nurse explained to him that this would pass in a few days, he was willing to accept the sleepiness. And it did pass. Within five days of starting his pain medicine, which was adjusted daily, Tom was free of pain at last.*

OPIOIDS ARE POWERFUL MEDICINES that are used alone or with nonopioids to alleviate moderate to severe pain, as well as breakthrough pain. Opioids are similar to natural substances (endorphins) produced by the body to control pain.

If your pain is not relieved by nonopioids alone, including opioids in your pain-control plan will usually give you the relief you need. Opioids may cause various side effects, most of which can be prevented or controlled.

In chapter 5, we introduced types of pain medications and listed their possible side effects. In this chapter, we'll revisit the side effects pain medications are most likely to cause and will provide practical strategies for preventing and managing these side effects. While not everyone has side effects from opioids, you can take an important step toward effectively managing any opioid side effects by keeping your doctor and nurse informed about how opioids affect your body.

Opioid Analgesic Side Effects

Opioid analgesics are often extremely effective in controlling cancer-related pain and discomfort, allowing you to go about your daily routine and enjoy activities in relative comfort. Yet the analgesics used to control pain can cause side effects—some mild and others more serious. These may include constipation, nausea, vomiting, a moderate decrease in the rate and depth of breathing, sedation, confusion, and delirium. In many cases, opioid-related side effects will ease or disappear after a few days as your body adjusts to the analgesics. But in some cases, the side effects may require medical attention.

Talk to your health care team about potential side effects before taking opioids. Many things can be done to manage side effects. In almost all cases, your doctor or nurse has many options to counteract and even completely eliminate them. Some measures may prevent side effects from occurring at all. If you suspect that you are experiencing side effects, let your doctor or nurse know right away, and ask for help. While you are taking opioid analgesics, communicate frequently with your health care team. Members of your health care team can help only if they know about your discomfort.

Digestive Tract Side Effects

Constipation
Constipation is the infrequent or difficult passage of hard feces (stool), which often causes pain and discomfort. This is the most common side effect of opioids. The likelihood that people taking opioids will have constipation is so high that most doctors will prescribe a treatment to prevent constipation with your first opioid dose. Even people taking

The extent to which constipation hinders your daily life is important to report because it indicates how severe the problem is and how quickly treatment should begin or if it should be increased.

When reporting your condition to your doctor or nurse, report all symptoms plus your bowel pattern and the day and type of your last bowel movement. For example, if the doctor or nurse knows there are stains of stool on your clothes or your rectal area feels full, they know the lower bowel needs to be evacuated and a laxative is required.

Contact your doctor or nurse if:
- you cannot move your bowels within one or two days after taking a laxative
- you have side effects of medication or other symptoms, such as persistent cramps, nausea, or vomiting
- your normal routine was one bowel movement a day and you haven't had one for three or four days, OR your normal routine was once every other day and you haven't had a bowel movement in four or five days
- you experience severe straining on the toilet or bedside commode
- you experience severe abdominal pain or your abdomen feels harder than normal and very full, OR you notice red blood around the outside of the stools or have problems with hemorrhoids
- you notice blood in or around the anal area or in stool
- constipation interferes with normal activities, such as walking or eating

weak opioids can develop constipation. The level of constipation can range from mild to severe. It can cause decreased appetite, bloating, and abdominal cramps. If left untreated, constipation can become a source of pain and discomfort and can lead to serious complications. In rare instances, constipation can be life-threatening. Fortunately, constipation is usually simple and easy to treat.

Because constipation and other digestive functions are highly personal, many people are embarrassed to talk about them with caregivers or medical personnel. Constipation can be prevented and controlled, but discussing the problem openly and honestly is essential so that those caring for you can treat and help relieve this uncomfortable and potentially dangerous condition.

CAUSES OF CONSTIPATION

Opioid pain medication, taken orally or by injection, is the most common cause of constipation among people with cancer. Opioids cause waste products to move more slowly along the intestinal tract, allowing more time for water to be absorbed by the intestines. The result is stool that becomes hard and difficult to pass. As the dose of opioids increases, constipation may increase. The constipation may not diminish over time unless some measures are taken to treat it.

A combination of factors often causes constipation in a person with cancer. Factors that contribute to constipation include:

- lack of activity
- general weakness
- ignoring the urge to have a bowel movement
- inadequate fluid intake
- changes in diet or a diet that contains too little fiber
- emotional stress, anxiety, or depression
- dehydration caused by fever and vomiting
- other medicines, such as chemotherapy drugs or antinausea medications

MANAGING CONSTIPATION

Patients who take opioid medicines usually begin a bowel program at the same time they start their opioid analgesics to prevent or at least minimize constipation. This may include dietary changes such as drinking more water and eating high-fiber foods and/or taking mild laxatives, stool softeners, suppositories, or enemas. People with cancer should avoid treating constipation without first seeking medical guidance.

In most cases, constipation can be controlled with laxatives and dietary changes. Mild laxatives contain naturally occurring bulk fiber, which causes stool to retain water and stimulates the bowels to move waste products more quickly toward the rectum. A commonly used mild laxative is senna (Senokot, Ex-Lax).

Stool softeners are often prescribed along with laxatives to draw moisture into the bowel, allowing stool to move more easily through the digestive tract. Laxatives may be combined with a stool softener such as docusate (Peri-Colace, Doxidan).

High-Fiber Foods

Keep in mind that people at risk for bowel obstruction should not eat diets high in fiber, including nuts, seeds, and the skins of raw fruits. Talk to your health care team about your situation and how you can best prevent and manage constipation.

Breads and Cereals	Serving Size	Dietary Fiber (grams)	Legumes	Serving Size	Dietary Fiber (grams)
Bran cereals	½ cup	3–13	Kidney beans*	½ cup	8
Popcorn	2 cups	5	Navy beans*	½ cup	9
Brown rice	½ cup	6			
Whole-wheat bread	1 slice	1–2	Fruit		
Wheat bran, raw	¼ cup	6			
			Apple with peel	1 medium	4
Vegetables			Banana	1 medium	2
			Blueberries	½ cup	2
Broccoli*	½ cup	4	Pear with skin	1 medium	5
Brussels sprouts*	½ cup	3	Prunes	3	3
Carrots	½ cup	2	Orange	1 medium	3
Corn	½ cup	5	Raisins	¼ cup	3
Green peas	½ cup	3	Strawberries	1 cup	3
Potato with skin	1 medium	3			

* These foods tend to cause gas.

© American Dietetic Association. 2000. *The Clinical Guide to Oncology Nutrition: Patient Education Materials.* Used with permission.

Consult your doctor before using any of these products to determine how much and how often you should take them. Doses of these medications should be gradually increased until they become effective.

Sometimes stronger laxatives, such as magnesium hydroxide (Milk of Magnesia) and magnesium citrate (MagCitrate) are needed to stimulate the bowels. The level of medication should be enough to help you produce bowel movements regularly—usually no more than two days apart. Note that patients with kidney disease should avoid laxatives containing magnesium (see the examples of stronger laxatives, above), and those with heart disease should avoid laxatives that contain sodium.

Adequate fluid intake is just as important as the use of laxatives. Doctors recommend eight to ten glasses of liquid daily, including water and fruit juices. Another remedy is to eat foods that contain high amounts of fiber (see the *High-Fiber Foods* section on page 147). The recommended intake of fiber is 25 to 35 grams a day. Regular exercise is also an important component of preventing constipation, if appropriate in your situation.

When constipation becomes severe and doesn't respond to laxatives and dietary adjustments, doctors may take more aggressive measures, such as suppositories or enemas, which may be appropriate for patients who are unable to keep food down and therefore cannot ingest adequate amounts of fiber through diet or laxatives. One option is a suppository inserted into the rectum to stimulate the lower bowel. (Suppositories should not be used for cancer patients who have low platelet or white blood cell counts because the suppository capsule may break small blood vessels in the rectal area, creating a risk of bleeding or infection.)

Another alternative for patients with severe constipation is an enema, which often brings immediate relief while causing minimal discomfort. Only one or two enemas are usually needed to relieve even severe constipation. Enema kits and commercial enema preparations, such as Fleet, can be purchased at pharmacies without a prescription.

Enema solutions containing mixtures of water and mineral oil or soap suds can be made at home. It is best to give an enema lying on your left side near a bathroom or with a portable commode next to the bed or couch. Before performing an enema at home, always check with a doctor or nurse. People who have lower colon surgery or other conditions involving the lower colon and rectum might not be able to have an enema.

Some people stop taking opioids without telling their doctors because constipation becomes so severe. This is not recommended since it will allow your pain to return. A better strategy is to inform your doctor or another member of your health care team about your condition so they can take steps to relieve both pain and constipation.

Fecal Impaction

Constipation that persists—whether because of insufficient treatment or because the person with cancer isn't following recommended methods of preventing or coping with constipation—can lead to a condition called fecal impaction. This occurs when pieces of dried stool become lodged in

Tips for Preventing and Managing Constipation

The best way to manage constipation is to prevent it. Following the steps below will minimize your risk of developing constipation when taking opioid medications. Talk to your health care team about your situation and how you can best prevent and manage constipation.

What to do:
- Drinking lots of fluids is the most important action you can take. Drink eight to ten cups of liquid each day (if allowed by your doctor). Try water, prune juice, warm juices, teas, and hot lemonade.
- Try to eat at the same times each day.
- Avoid liquids that contain caffeine.
- Eat foods high in fiber, such as uncooked fruits (with the skin on), vegetables, whole grain breads and cereals, fresh raw fruits with skins and seeds, dates, apricots, prunes, and nuts.
- Add one or two tablespoons of unprocessed bran to your food. This adds bulk and stimulates bowel movements. Keep a shaker of bran handy at mealtimes to make it easy to sprinkle on foods.
- Avoid foods and beverages that cause gas such as cabbage, broccoli, cauliflower, cucumbers, dried beans, peas, onions, and carbonated drinks.
- Get as much exercise as you can, even if that means only walking a very short distance.
- Try to have a bowel movement whenever you have the urge.
- Use stool softeners or laxatives only as instructed by your doctor or nurse.
- Use a rectal suppository only after checking with your doctor or nurse.
- If you are confined to bed, try to use the toilet or bedside commode when you have a bowel movement, even if that is the only time you get out of bed.
- Use an enema to provide immediate relief from constipation, but first check with the doctor or nurse. Enemas should be the last step for relieving constipation. They evacuate the lower bowel and help the upper bowel move as well.

Do not:
- strain or use extreme force when trying to move your bowels
- use over-the-counter laxatives or enemas unless first discussed with your doctor
- eat foods that can cause constipation, such as chocolate, cheese, eggs, and refined grain products (cakes, cookies, donuts, etc.)
- use laxatives and enemas if you have a low white blood count or low platelet count

the rectum or intestines and block the ability of the gastrointestinal system to empty. Left untreated, fecal impaction can be dangerous. If it is not diagnosed and if patients do not continue to take strong laxatives, the bowel may rupture behind the impaction.

Most fecal impactions occur in the rectum. The most common treatment is for the doctor or nurse to manually remove the stool with a gloved finger, then wash the area with an enema. The procedure may be painful and an anesthetic or sedative may be necessary for the patient's comfort. Fecal impaction that occurs higher in the colon can usually be eliminated with enemas.

Elderly patients, especially those who are easily confused, may not know that they have fecal impaction because the condition may cause no early symptoms except lack of bowel movements. Patients may first complain of pressure in the abdomen caused by the blockage. Diarrhea may even occur as loose stool and mucus seeps around the blockage and leaks from the rectum. This can cause skin breakdown, infections of the urinary tract, total bowel obstruction, and bacterial infection from the intestines.

Nausea and Vomiting

Nausea is an extremely unpleasant condition that can cause minimal difficulties or may cause a great deal of suffering. It can leave people weak and unable to carry out normal routines. People with severe nausea often find that they cannot even get out of bed. Vomiting often accompanies nausea.

Frequent nausea and vomiting can also lead to serious complications, such as dehydration or breathing in food or liquids. In addition, people suffering from nausea typically have no desire to eat, which may make them weaker.

Approximately one-third of all patients who take opioids will experience some degree of nausea. However, the body usually becomes tolerant to opioid-caused nausea after a few days and the side effects disappear.

CAUSES OF NAUSEA AND VOMITING

Opioids produce nausea and vomiting by stimulating the vomiting center in the brain and by affecting the gastrointestinal (GI) tract. Constipation, which is almost always a side effect of opioids, can also lead to nausea.

Sometimes patients who experience nausea when first starting their opioid medication think they are "allergic" to the medicine. Some people think they are allergic to opioids if they experience nausea. Nausea and vomiting alone usually are not allergic responses. But a rash or itching along with nausea and vomiting may be an allergic reaction. If this occurs, stop taking the medicine and tell your doctor at once.

Nonsteroidal anti-inflammatory drugs (NSAIDs) can also cause nausea and vomiting in some patients. When taken for a long period of time, NSAIDs irritate the stomach lining and can also cause ulcer-like symptoms. Other sources of cancer-related nausea include tumors that partially or completely block the intestinal tract and injury to abdominal tissue and kidneys from radiation therapy. Nausea may also result from tumors in the brain or those that have spread from their original site to other parts of the body. Nausea and vomiting are also two of the most common side effects of chemotherapy.

Nausea and vomiting caused by opioids will usually disappear after you take them for a few days. Following the tips below may help you cope with nausea in the meantime:

- Stay in bed for an hour or so after you take your medicine if you feel nauseous when you walk around. This type of nausea is like motion sickness, and over-the-counter medicines such as meclizine (Antivert, Dramamine II) or dimenhydrinate (Dramamine) may help. Check with your doctor or nurse before taking these medicines.
- If pain itself is the cause of the nausea, using opioids to relieve the pain usually makes the nausea go away.
- Antinausea medicines that relieve nausea can sometimes be prescribed.
- Ask your doctor or nurse if the cancer, some other medical condition, or other medicine you are taking such as steroids, anticancer drugs, or aspirin might be causing your nausea. Constipation may also contribute to nausea.

MANAGING NAUSEA AND VOMITING

The good news is that nausea and vomiting related to opioid analgesics is usually short-lived and can almost always be relieved with medications called antiemetics. Fortunately, doctors have a number of antiemetics at their disposal. Different antiemetics work for different people, and it may be necessary to try more than one before you get relief. Continue to work with your doctor and nurse to find the medicine that works best for you.

Routine preventive use of antinausea medicines may not be necessary, but your doctor may make these medicines available to you in case you need them. Milder antinausea medicines, such as prochlorperazine (Compazine) or metoclopramide (Reglan), will usually relieve nausea for those taking opioids for the first time. If nausea continues when you take milder antinausea medicines as needed, your doctor may recommend taking antinausea medicines on a regular schedule. If nausea persists for more than one week, the doctor will usually reconsider the cause of the nausea. If the nausea is related to the opioid, then the doctor may:

- recommend a different opioid medicine
- add an adjuvant analgesic in order to reduce the dose of opioid
- give you a stronger antinausea medicine

Central Nervous System Side Effects

Respiratory Depression

Respiratory depression is slow, shallow breathing. (Respiratory depression is different than shortness of breath, which is difficulty getting one's breath. Sometimes people with lung problems that cause shortness of breath, such as pneumonia or emphysema, may be given an opioid to relieve this symptom.) Many people think that respiratory depression is a very common effect of opioids. It is not common, but when it does occur, it causes patients and families a great deal of anxiety. It is potentially the most serious of all the side effects related to opioid analgesics.

Patients who have never taken opioids before and those who may have significant lung disease are most likely to experience respiratory depression. It is also less likely to occur when patients have normal liver and kidney function.

Respiratory depression is related to the effect of the opioids on the central nervous system. This opioid side effect is very unusual when the opioid dose prescribed is appropriate to the degree of pain. The risk of opioid-caused respiratory depression decreases over time. As a result, opioid analgesics can be used to treat cancer pain without significant risk of respiratory depression. Respiratory depression from opioid analgesics that is not resolved with the passage of time can usually be controlled with medication. If you are taking opioids, call your doctor immediately if you experience slow breathing or very shallow breathing (short breaths that don't take in much air).

Sedation

Opioids may also cause sedation, or a drowsy feeling. This drowsiness can lower the quality of life for people so that they limit the opioids they take, even though they are in pain.

When to Notify Your Health Care Team about Respiratory Depression

You or your caregivers should contact your doctor or nurse if:
- your family or caregiver notices slow breathing
- your skin looks pale or takes on a bluish color
- your skin feels cold and clammy
- your family cannot awaken you or has difficulty arousing you
- you experience any confusion

Tips for Managing Respiratory Depression

- Remain calm.
- Do not stop taking your opioid medicines without first talking with your doctor.
- Do not increase your opioid therapy without your doctor's advice.
- Notify your doctor if you are taking any medicines that he or she might not know about (including tranquilizers and other sedatives, herbs, vitamins, or any other supplements).

Beginning opioid therapy for the first time or taking significantly more opioids at the recommendation of your doctor can cause you to feel drowsy until your body adjusts to the opioid. This can take a few days or a week.

CAUSES OF SEDATION

Sedation is caused by the effects of opioids on the central nervous system. More specifically, factors that can cause sedation include an imbalance of chemicals in the blood (for example, sodium or calcium) and other medicines that could cause sedation, such as sedatives, tranquilizers, tricyclic antidepressants, and some other types of antidepressants.

If you have not been sleeping—for example, because of pain—what may seem like sedation related to opioids might actually be a natural effect of pain relief. This natural "catching up" on sleep may be confused with over-sedation.

MANAGING SEDATION

Usually sedation will subside within several days. If the drowsy feeling persists, your health care team will usually reduce the dose of each opioid while increasing the dose frequency. Your doctor might switch you to another opioid or opt for long-acting or sustained-release opioids, which can decrease sedation. These medicines may not meet your changing pain needs, so they might be combined with short-acting opioids that can be used as "rescue" therapy for breakthrough pain. A psychostimulant may be used to decrease sedation while allowing you to take a high enough dose of opioids to relieve your pain.

When to Notify Your Health Care Team about Sedation

Contact your doctor or nurse if:
- sedation lasts more than one week
- your family cannot rouse you
- you are concerned about the amount of time you are sleeping
- any confusion occurs
- there is a decrease in your rate of breathing

- It is often best to avoid driving for two weeks after starting opioids or increasing the dose of opioids.
- Do not confuse "catching up" on sleep with sedation.
- Notify your doctor if you are taking any medicines that he or she might not know about (including herbs, vitamins, or any other supplements).

Confusion and Delirium

The potential opioid side effects of confusion and delirium may be frightening for people with cancer and their families and caregivers. Delirium is characterized by a change in mental function and a change in level of consciousness that accompanies less of an ability to focus attention or shift attention. These changes may develop within a short time and fluctuate throughout the day. Symptoms include difficulty sleeping, nightmares, irritability, anxiety, difficulty concentrating, attention deficits, memory disturbances, and abnormal psychomotor behavior, such as picking at bed covers.

Mild brain function impairment is common after starting opioids or increasing a dose. However, major brain impairment is usually temporary in most patients, lasting from a few days to one to two weeks.

The first manifestation of delirium may be something as mild as nightmares, anxiety, insomnia, or irritability, but can progress rapidly to something as severe as hallucinations. Be aware of these symptoms and talk to your health care team if you, your family members, or your caregiver notice them; if delirium is not identified as such, additional medication may be recommended to alleviate the symptoms and may worsen the delirium.

CAUSES OF CONFUSION AND DELIRIUM

Confusion and delirium may result from the effect of opioids on the central nervous system, but often involve other factors as well. Persistent confusion may be due to opioid use alone, but it is usually related to a combined effect of the opioid and other factors, such as other medications, fluid and electrolyte imbalances, tumors affecting the brain or central nervous system, major organ problems, or reduced oxygen intake.

MANAGING CONFUSION AND DELIRIUM

Your doctor will evaluate the cause or causes of confusion and delirium, which often involve multiple factors. If the cause is the opioid analgesic, lowering the dose of the opioid may resolve the side effect. In other cases, the opioid may need to be changed. Other medicines that could be contributing to the delirium (sleeping aids, tranquilizers, anxiolytics, and antihistamines, which may cause side effects that may contribute to the delirium) will be stopped and your health care team will review your

---

When to Notify Your Health Care Team about Confusion and Delirium

Contact your doctor or nurse if:
- you, your family members, or your caregiver notice that you are having any symptoms of delirium
- you are confused
- you are having any other symptoms
- you are taking any medicines that your doctor might not know about (including herbs, vitamins, or any other supplements)
- you have a fever, chills, or other symptom of infection

Tips for Managing Delirium

- Surround yourself with familiar family, friends, objects, and sounds.
- Have a family member or friend stay with you if delirium occurs.
- Have someone orient you to time, place, and date several times each day.
- Have someone notify your doctor if symptoms increase or change.
- Notify your doctor if you are taking any medicines that he or she might not know about (including herbs, vitamins, or any other supplements).

recent cancer treatment. Many doctors will ask for an evaluation by a psychiatrist to be certain of the underlying cause. Surrounding yourself with familiar people, objects, and sounds and being made aware of time, place, and date on a frequent basis may help you cope. Haloperidol (Haldol) or other related medications, such as olanzapine (Zyprexa) and clozapine (Clorazil), may help manage delirium.

CHAPTER 9

Cancer Pain in Specific Groups

*J*uan had colorectal cancer that had spread to his bones. He had fallen and broken a bone in his left arm, but he never asked for pain medicine. His wife knew he must be in pain. But when anyone from the health care team asked him about his pain, he replied that he did not need any medicine. His wife explained that Juan came from a family in which the man was the ruler and provider of the house. He did not have time to attend to the children, did not have time for illness, and never showed emotions. This was the way he lived; this was his culture.

FORTUNATELY, THERE IS NO NEED TO SUFFER IN SILENCE. No matter what your background or age is, you have many options for pain relief. Proper treatment for cancer pain generally follows established principles and guidelines designed to match pain-relief treatments with the severity of pain while keeping patients as alert, comfortable, and functional as possible.

As we have discussed, treatments for pain include a variety of medications, therapies, and nondrug treatments. While these methods are appropriate for treating most cases of cancer pain, some patient populations have special considerations that may alter pain-management strategies. These groups include infants and children, the elderly, patients with a history of substance abuse, patients from diverse cultures, and those who are critically ill.

Children and Cancer Pain

Advances in recent years have greatly improved our knowledge about the effectiveness of cancer treatment in children. But neither the causes nor the treatment of cancer pain in children are as well studied or as well understood as they are for adults.

Pain in children should be taken seriously and treated aggressively by doctors, nurses, and caregivers. Yet too often children are not provided with adequate pain relief because of mistaken ideas about how they experience and cope with pain. Some health care professionals still incorrectly believe that the nature and causes of cancer-related pain among children are the same as for adults, that identical pain-relief strategies apply, or that pain control is less important for children than for adults.

At one time, many doctors and other health care professionals accepted the notion that children, especially infants, experienced less pain than adults. Another common misconception among medical professionals has been that children are more susceptible to dependence on medication and side effects caused by opioids. These medications effectively reduce pain regardless of a patient's age, and addiction is uncommon. Opioids can even be used safely in very young infants. (Newborns are more prone to the potential side effect of respiratory depression than older children, however.) Regardless of their age, children are able to feel and suffer from pain. Children do not recover from pain any faster than adults do. They form and remember clear associations between pain and its causes.

Children struggle with cancer and cancer pain, but they may also face a sense of helplessness as they are shuttled to and from unfamiliar environments for strangers to examine them, question them (if they are old enough to talk), poke and prod them, and conduct tests or procedures that may cause additional pain. Children may not understand the reasons tests or procedures are necessary and may feel fear, anxiety, and discomfort. Parents and health care professionals need to take special measures to comfort children before, during, and after tests or treatments and to continually reassure them that their medical care is essential to help them get better.

Sources of Cancer-Related Pain among Children

Cancer is relatively rare among children, accounting for less than one percent of all malignancies. However, many of these children with cancer suffer disease-related pain, which can be severe. Some research even suggests that children with cancer pain may be more sensitive to additional pain.

A child's experience of cancer pain is likely to be very different from that of an adult, primarily because the source of their pain usually differs. In adults, pain often develops when solid tumors grow and press on pain sensitive tissue, compress nerves, or block hollow organs. Adults' tumors spread to other parts of the body, where they invade other body organs and cause pain. Solid tumors are less common in children. Childhood cancers are more commonly found in the bloodstream or lymphatic system. Leukemia (cancers of the blood or blood-forming organs) and lymphoma (cancer of the lymphatic system) respond quickly to treatment. Only later, if they do recur, would these cancers potentially cause cancer-related pain.

About 80 percent of children report that they experience pain caused by cancer treatment, and that diagnostic procedures cause them pain. For relatively common childhood cancers, such as leukemia, painful diagnostic procedures may need to be performed frequently. For example, children with leukemia require spinal taps, during which a needle is inserted into the spine to remove spinal fluid (see chapter 1). Other examples of potentially painful diagnostic tests include bone marrow biopsies and drawing blood for blood tests.

In addition to diagnostic procedures, clinical procedures may also be sources of pain for children with cancer. With surgery, there is always acute incisional pain for a few to several days. Infections can also cause pain. Additionally, receiving chemotherapy or radiation can cause mouth sores, sore throat, abdominal cramping with diarrhea or constipation, tingling and prickly sensations in hands and feet, muscle cramps, and joint pain in children.

When painful tests and treatment procedures must be repeated throughout the cancer treatment experience, children are exposed to predictable episodes of pain that they may dread (see *Anticipating Pain*, below). Child life specialists—experts with master's degrees in child development—can be invaluable in helping children and their parents through these procedures. Child life specialists are typically available at major medical centers.

Anticipating Pain

Painful experiences at the hospital or doctor's office often stand out in a child's memory and can lead to anticipatory pain and distress well before the next procedure or test. Since most children are afraid of needles and virtually all of them have received injections, they may become anxious and fearful while waiting for any test or procedure that involves needles. Even when tests cause no physical pain—such as x-rays, CT scans, or MRIs—scheduled procedures may still cause worry and fear. Just the anticipation of returning to the hospital may generate associations with previous painful experiences.

Tests and procedures that may feel insignificant and routine to adults—such as blood draws—can be traumatic for children and may create lasting emotional impressions. Parents and health care professionals should not forget that "minor" medical treatment can create tremendous anxiety and fear among children. These powerful emotions may translate into less cooperation from children.

Before any visit to the doctor, parents should explain in age-appropriate language the reason for the visit and what to expect. All children old enough to talk should be counseled and reassured by caregivers before, during, and after any test or procedure, regardless of whether or not it will cause pain. Whenever possible, one or both parents should be at their child's side throughout procedures or tests.

Pain Assessment in Children

The criteria for evaluating children's pain are similar to those used for adults. Initial pain assessments typically consist of a comprehensive history and physical examination, including questions about the type, location, and severity of pain and the steps parents have taken to control it. Yet evaluating children often presents unique challenges, especially if patients are too young to communicate verbally.

The Challenge of Communication

The capacity of children to communicate varies considerably. As they grow, their ability to verbally communicate information about their pain increases. By the age of six, many children can describe pain severity, location, duration, and type. Some may be evaluated with the same pain scales used with adults (see chapter 4).

Some pain scales are used specifically for children. For example, the "Oucher" scale shows a measure from 0 to 100 and six photographs of a four year old's face displaying different expressions, each corresponding to a different level of pain intensity. Other child-oriented pain scales match different colors to pain intensity or use poker chips to represent "pieces of hurt." When using these scales, the evaluator asks children how many chips their pain has. For teenagers, a list of words describing types of pain may be useful.

Some children are quite capable of telling doctors, nurses, and caregivers where and how much they hurt. Some can describe various characteristics of their pain, discriminate among different types of pain sensations, report how their pain changes throughout the day, and link specific activities that cause increased or decreased pain. Others have great difficulty talking about their sensations.

Observing Behavior to Gauge Pain

Pain behaviors change as children develop. For example, an infant may respond to pain with generalized movements, changes in facial expressions, and crying, whereas toddlers can signal the location of their pain, and older children are generally capable of describing their pain in some detail, or at least indicating pain severity from a rating scale.

Infants and very young children cannot communicate the location or intensity of their pain, which makes pain assessment particularly challenging. The only way infants express pain is to cry, but this behavior may also signal hunger or a wet diaper rather than pain. Doctors often must judge pain intensity from a child's behavior and from physiological signs, such as breathing rate, heart rate, and palm sweating, as well as from parents' reports. Parents should carefully observe a child, paying particular attention to facial expressions, unusual behavior, and any other signs that may indicate pain.

Even when parents watch a young child to try to gauge pain, they may find it difficult to gauge pain levels. Some children, even those capable of talking, may not complain or cry, which makes pain assessment even more difficult. Silence in the presence of pain may indicate that a child has given up hope and requires emotional support from caregivers and their health care team. Parents and health care professionals must watch for other signs of pain, discomfort, or distress.

Older children may cry not just as a result of pain, but also because they are afraid or anxious about upcoming tests or procedures. For doctors, nurses, and caregivers, making the distinction between an upset child and a child in pain can be difficult. In either case, a child in distress requires attention. *When children appear to be in pain, they should be treated as if they are, even when parents or doctors are unsure.*

Managing Cancer Pain in Children

Acute pain in children caused by procedures and tests can be minimized using a combination of drug therapy, nondrug pain-relief techniques, and lots of reassurance from parents and the medical staff. For example, a child undergoing a spinal tap to collect spinal fluid may benefit from a detailed explanation of what to expect, a local anesthetic cream over the puncture site, relaxation and distraction, an antianxiety medicine, and a strong, short-acting analgesic. Some health care professionals advise parents to discuss the procedure with their child to build trust and further explain why their treatment is so important.

The choices of pain treatments vary, depending on the amount of pain expected during a procedure as well as an individual child's level of anxiety or fear. For more invasive procedures, such as bone marrow sampling, a general anesthetic may be necessary to make the child unconscious during the test.

Another pain-control technique specially designed for children is conscious sedation, in which just enough medication is given (preferably by mouth) to decrease pain caused by procedures or tests. Conscious sedation allows children to remain conscious enough to respond to voice commands and questions.

Therapy with Pain Medicines

The principles of pain control for children are similar to those applied to adults. Chronic pain caused by cancer can usually be controlled with oral pain medications, including acetaminophen, NSAIDs, and opioid analgesics. Most analgesic medications used for adults work well for children when doses are adjusted for their age and body weight. Two NSAIDs—tolmetin (Tolectin) and naproxen (Aleve)—are specifically approved by the U.S. Food and Drug Administration for treating children. NSAIDs are particularly effective for treating mild to moderate pain caused by inflammation or bone tumors. However, these medications should not be prescribed for children who are at risk for internal bleeding or for children who need to be monitored for fever during chemotherapy treatments. Children should not receive aspirin because it increases the risk of Reye's Syndrome, a potentially serious and life-limiting condition. Your doctor will tell you if your child is old enough to take aspirin.

Opioids are the mainstay of treatment for moderate to severe pain in children just as they are for adult patients. Doctors may also prescribe antidepressants, stimulants, and corticosteroids to enhance children's pain relief. For children with continuous pain, pain medications should be administered on a strict schedule around the clock, not just as needed, to ensure that sufficient levels of analgesics remain in the bloodstream throughout the day. Children should also have extra doses of pain medication ("breakthrough" or "rescue" medications) available to them for when pain flares up or to be used before taking part in activities expected to increase pain. If children whose cancer has spread to the bone experience increased pain when they move, for example, they should have pain medications available to take before they are physically active.

Ideally, pain medications are given orally to children to avoid pain caused by needle sticks. (Some medicines can be crushed and placed in food or drinks.) Young children cannot connect the pain of injection with future relief, and many would rather live with their pain than get injections. When injections are necessary, doctors or nurses can apply an anesthetic cream over the injection site to minimize pain. If children refuse to take medicines by mouth, alternatives include opioid patches, suppositories, and also subcutaneously or intravenously administered pain medications, both of which children can receive at home. Refusal to take medications orally may mean that children are exercising the last bit of control they have during a process about which they feel helpless.

Other Medical Approaches to Pain Management

Doctors rarely use nerve blocks or surgical procedures to relieve a child's pain. But these techniques work well when they are necessary. In fact, nerve blocks and morphine given into the epidural space of the spine have been used successfully in very young babies. Some pain-control options that are suitable for adults are inappropriate for children. For example, regional anesthesia is not a reasonable solution for most children because their pain often occurs across a large area of the body and is hard to pinpoint.

As with adults, the risk of dependence or addiction among children is extremely low and should not prevent doctors from prescribing opioids. Some doctors still mistakenly believe that opioids should not be prescribed to young children. In most cases, weak and strong opioids can be combined with other medications for adequate pain relief.

Some types of constant pain are managed better by continued opioid infusion, even for children who are at home. This method of medication delivery requires a doctor to surgically place a catheter just under the skin and into a large vein (see chapter 5). A special pump attached to the catheter dispenses medications automatically at regular intervals. The technique eliminates the need for repeated injections. Children as young as five have been taught to use patient-controlled analgesia—they decide when intravenous medications are needed and push a button to cause the medicine to flow through the catheter into their bloodstream.

Nondrug Techniques of Pain Relief

Many of the same nondrug pain-relief methods that have proven to be effective for adults can be altered appropriately to provide relief for children (see chapter 7). Such techniques include biofeedback, relaxation therapy, distraction, desensitization, hypnosis, imagery, and psychological counseling for both children with cancer and their families. Children are particularly responsive to distraction because it involves imagination and "pretending." Children also respond well to music and being rocked, massaged, or stroked during painful periods. Applying heat or cold to sensitive areas can also be effective. Although nondrug techniques cannot eliminate pain completely, they often reduce pain to some extent and may enhance the effects of medication.

Reassurance and Support

Providing realistic reassurance and comfort to children before their very first cancer-related procedure helps reduce anxiety and fear before and during future procedures. Loved ones should be present before, during, and after treatment to offer reassurance and help the child calm down and relax. Research shows that children having procedures greatly benefit from having a loved one present to provide a sense of security and lessen fears of abandonment.

Adults should remain calm during tests and procedures, since children take their cues from adults. An adult who appears nervous or fearful will have a far more difficult time settling down a child than one who appears relaxed and confident. Often, simply offering factual information about a procedure is an effective strategy because it returns some sense of control and realistic expectations to a child. Having a greater sense of control can reduce some of the feelings of helplessness associated with having cancer and undergoing painful procedures. Distractions such as books or toys may also be useful to lower anxiety and pass the time while waiting for a procedure. If the child is old enough to understand, parents should explain in detail what to expect during the upcoming treatment. A child's fantasies are often worse than reality.

During diagnostic and therapeutic procedures, children should have adequate privacy. Health care professionals should ensure that they feel comfortable and secure. Parents can help by bringing familiar items from home, such as favorite toys, pictures, books, or stuffed animals. Music, video games, and television are also effective distractions for children. For hospitalized children, the health care team and parents or caregivers may want to schedule a tour of the hospital, and may want to designate "safe times" during which the child can rest assured that no procedures or tests will be performed. Talk to other children and their parents or caregivers to see what worked for them.

Cancer Pain in the Elderly Person

Older people who have cancer deserve thorough and aggressive pain management. Yet misconceptions and inappropriate beliefs about how this group experiences and copes with pain often impede appropriate care. According to pain-control guidelines issued by the government, the elderly are at risk for undertreated cancer pain. Increased research into pain and the elderly is helping to emphasize the management of pain for older persons.

Pain is extremely common among older people, and it often goes undetected. An estimated 25 to 50 percent of elderly people have chronic pain problems. For nursing home residents, it is estimated that 45 to 80 percent have substantial pain that is untreated. This group often requires special considerations because of physiological and psychological changes that occur with aging.

Many people assume that increased pain is a normal part of the aging process—a condition to be endured without complaint. Some health care professionals wrongly believe that older people are less sensitive to pain and that they cannot tolerate opioid pain medications well. While it is true that older adults are likely to experience more chronic pain than younger ones, particularly in the muscles and joints, there is no reason to ignore frequent pain or leave it untreated.

Health care professionals should pursue pain management aggressively for elderly patients. Caregivers or people with cancer who feel that their reports of pain do not get adequate attention should speak frankly with a doctor or nurse on the health care team about reducing their pain.

Pain Assessment in Elderly Patients

Accurately assessing pain among elderly patients poses some unique challenges. Older people tend to understate the amount of pain they experience and may need to be prompted several times before they provide an accurate description of the severity and type of their pain. Some older patients are reluctant to complain about pain or to display behaviors that indicate they are in pain, possibly because older individuals often live with one or more conditions that cause pain, such as arthritis, so they do not pay particular attention to new pain beyond considering it yet another burden of aging they must endure. Assessment of cancer-related pain in the elderly is difficult for health professionals because of other factors that cause pain, and because patients may wait until pain becomes severe before they visit a doctor.

Some degree of mental impairment is present in an estimated five percent of patients 65 years and older and in more than 20 percent of those older than 80 years. Patients with mental impairment, such as Alzheimer's disease, may be unable to discuss their pain or provide adequate information to doctors or nurses. They may not remember when their pain starts, how severe it becomes, or what measures bring relief. Their reports of pain may change often and quickly. As a result, elderly patients often require pain assessments more frequently than younger ones. Patients with diminished mental functioning or who have difficulty verbalizing thoughts may be better able to describe their pain through the use of simplified pain scales, such as a faces scale (see chapter 4 for more information about pain scales).

Older patients may have hearing and vision difficulties, making communication with caregivers and medical personnel more difficult. And pain and pain treatment may make elderly patients unable to accurately describe their condition because both pain and opioids may dull a person's mental ability and decrease alertness.

Doctors and nurses can learn important information by assessing pain before and after a patient receives analgesics to determine the effectiveness of treatment. But when treating elderly patients who do not communicate well, doctors might have to rely on caregivers to observe behavioral changes that signal whether pain has decreased, remained constant, or increased after therapy.

Managing Cancer Pain in the Elderly Person

Strategies for managing pain in elderly people with cancer follow the same fundamental principles used for treating younger adults. Yet misconceptions about pain in older patients often lead to inadequate treatment.

The cornerstone of treatment for cancer pain among elderly patients is drug therapy, just as it is for younger patients. Acetaminophen, aspirin,

NSAIDs, and opioids should be administered in doses that match the severity and type of pain, as outlined in chapter 5. Treatment may be supplemented with adjuvant medications, such as antianxiety medications, antidepressants, and steroids. But some important considerations must be kept in mind when treating elderly patients with medications.

Most pain medications are processed (metabolized) by the liver and kidneys. In elderly people, these and other organs tend to function less efficiently and to be more dramatically affected by medications. In addition, the elderly bodies generally have less water and muscle mass and more body fat than those of younger adults. Therefore older patients may not tolerate doses of analgesics as well as younger ones, and determining the most effective dose can be a challenge for doctors. NSAIDs may cause more side effects among elderly patients than in younger ones, including high blood pressure, kidney problems, dizziness, confusion, and excessive salt and water retention. Elderly patients who begin taking NSAIDs should be watched closely to ensure good kidney function.

An advantage to lower drug tolerance among the elderly is that lower doses often achieve adequate pain relief and last longer. Therefore, doctors usually begin pain medications at lower doses for elderly people with cancer and increase them more gradually than they would for younger patients. This precaution not only decreases the chances for medication-related side effects, but also lessens the risk of adverse reactions caused by mixing pain medicines with other medicines patients may already be taking, which can cause similar side effects.

Some doctors still believe that elderly patients shouldn't receive opioids, or only prescribe them at very low doses for the elderly. The result is often inadequate pain relief. Older people are more sensitive to the effects of opioids, but these medications should play a very important role in cancer pain relief, regardless of a patient's age. Elderly patients are likely to experience grogginess and sedation when opioid treatment begins; however, these side effects usually diminish shortly after the start of drug therapy. The elderly may also experience slowed breathing, but this does not mean opioid therapy should be discontinued. Opioids may also cause nausea and vomiting, which can be relieved with appropriate antinausea medications. To reduce constipation associated with opioids, doctors usually prescribe laxatives as soon as a patient begins taking opioids (see chapter 8). Because older individuals are usually less physically active, drink less fluid, and are more likely to take other medications that cause constipation than younger people, laxatives are particularly important factors in keeping patients comfortable.

For elderly patients who cannot take medications orally, alternate routes of drug delivery are available, including suppositories and subcu-taneously and intravenously administered medications. Chemical and surgical nerve blocks are just as effective in elderly patients as they are in younger ones, but older patients may not tolerate the side effects of these procedures very well and may require longer recovery periods. Patient-controlled analgesia is useful for some elderly patients, but should be closely monitored by the health care team or caregivers at home. (See chapter 5 for more information about drug delivery methods and pain relief.)

Elderly patients often take multiple medications to treat other conditions in addition to cancer. As more medications are added to the list, the risk of adverse and potentially dangerous drug interactions increases. To minimize the threat of drug interactions, inform doctors of all the medications you are taking, including any vitamins or herbal preparations.

Elderly patients or their caregivers should maintain regular and frequent contact with members of the health care team to closely monitor drug effectiveness and drug-related side effects, and to make changes to the program as needed. Their pain should be reassessed whenever they move to a new setting, such as from the hospital to home, or when changes are made to the pain therapy program.

> ## *Family Members Can Help*
>
> Family members are often crucial to successfully managing pain in elderly patients. Caregivers, who may be elderly themselves, often assume significant burdens when caring for an elderly cancer patient. They must be sure that the patient takes the correct pain medicine on time and at the prescribed dose, monitor the patient for changes in pain status (such as the emergence of breakthrough pain), and keep in touch with members of the health care team. This can be a demanding and exhausting responsibility. Some caregivers may require the assistance of home nursing, home hospice services, home health aides, and volunteers (see the *Resources* section) to assume some of their duties, provide periodic rests, and ease their physical and psychological stress.

Emotional and Psychological Issues
Related to Pain in the Elderly

Elderly patients require a significant amount of emotional support to deal with cancer and its treatment. If symptoms of cancer, including pain, are not addressed, older patients are more likely than others to suffer chronic pain, depression, sleep disturbances, impaired ability to walk, falls, slow rehabilitation, problems caused by taking multiple medications, mental impairment, and malnutrition.

A high number of patients who suffer from chronic pain also experience depression and anxiety at some time during cancer treatment. As discussed earlier, depression often causes patients to experience greater pain (see chapter 2 for more information). An elderly person with cancer should talk to the health care team about his or her emotional state so the plan for pain management can take into account any depression or anxiety. (The health care team will also consider the physical and psychological effects of pain medications and other treatments.)

When properly planned and carried out, pain therapy for the elderly can greatly reduce and even eliminate pain and discomfort, which frees elderly people with cancer to pursue daily activities and enjoy greatly improved quality of life.

Treatment Issues for People with a History of Substance Abuse

Cancer patients who have a history of alcohol or drug abuse require special attention when they need drug therapy to relieve pain. In order to ensure effective and safe treatment, honesty is essential; it's important to inform doctors, other members of the health care team, and caregivers if you have any history of substance abuse or have a current issue of substance abuse. People with cancer always serve their own best interests by being candid with their health care team. If you hold back information about current or past drug abuse, you risk getting medication doses that are too low to relieve pain.

Some doctors are reluctant to prescribe opioids to patients who abuse or have abused drugs in the past, fearing that they will become addicted. As discussed earlier, the risk of addiction from cancer pain medication in the general population is extremely low, affecting less than one percent of patients who have no history of substance abuse (see chapter 5). Although the risk increases substantially among those who have abused drugs or alcohol, this does not mean that medications, even strong opioids such as morphine, should be withheld from cancer patients in pain. Doctors must weigh the pain-relieving benefits of drug therapy against the risks of dependence for each patient.

One strategy to reduce the chances of becoming addicted to pain medications is to first rely on medications such as NSAIDs and steroids—which are not habit-forming—for mild to moderate pain. Patients who have had substance abuse problems, like any other patients, must communicate frequently with their health care team to let them know if pain-relief measures are effective. If they need stronger medications to control pain, doctors will insist that drugs be taken precisely as prescribed—on time and at the correct dosage—and may also ask patients to keep pain medication diaries to ensure that they adhere to the drug therapy plan. Caregivers can play an important role by supervising the use and dosage of opioids to prevent abuse.

Health professionals with experience treating people in pain have reported that though a small number of patients lie about pain levels so that they can get higher drug doses, most take medicines reliably and in correct amounts. Patients who use their pain medications improperly or make awkward excuses about why their prescriptions run low ahead of schedule risk losing their doctors' trust and may not receive adequate pain control in the future. If prescribed medications meet pain-relief needs and are used as prescribed, there should be no need for early refills. Doctors may choose to prescribe only a week's worth of pain medication at a time to reduce the chances that patients will take extra opioids. Talking to your health care team regularly and in detail about your pain intensity, pain medication doses, and pain relief will help ensure that your pain-relief needs are clear and will demonstrate that you are following the plan.

Doctors may prescribe long-acting opioids to be taken on a regular schedule rather than prescribing short-acting medications "as needed." Longer-acting opioids provide more consistent pain relief and tend not to produce "highs" associated with the shorter-acting medications. Patients who are recovered addicts may worry about starting therapy with medications that can potentially lead to dependence. The health care team can provide these patients with reassurance and close supervision during drug therapy.

Cancer patients with a history of substance abuse may find it helpful to consult medical professionals who are knowledgeable about both cancer pain and drug dependence. Doctors may advise patients who are at home to work with psychiatric and substance abuse counselors to ensure that they stick to prescribed drug therapy and prevent drug abuse. Substance abusers may also require more psychological counseling for mental health problems than other patients.

Culturally Diverse Groups

Cultural background has a powerful influence on how people react to and cope with pain and illness. It often affects how patients express and rate pain, what significance pain has, how a person normally copes with pain, how acceptable it is to have others present during doctor visits, and what traditional or folk remedies a patient uses or has used in the past.

In some cultures, the vocal expression of pain is considered weak behavior, whereas enduring pain is considered a sign of strength. Men in particular may be expected to endure pain and discomfort without complaining. It cannot be assumed that people who don't talk about pain aren't suffering or won't benefit from pain therapy. People in other cultural groups may be more vocal about their pain and think nothing of displaying their discomfort as a way to bring relief, and they may even demand pain control. Expressions of crying and moaning can be ways of attempting to relieve pain and may not accurately reflect the severity of distress. In some cultural traditions, people believe that pain is the result of supernatural powers, fate, punishment for previous deeds, evil spirits, or witchcraft, and that it is closely associated with death. To some patients, the pain may be as significant as the illness itself.

To provide the best care, health professionals must consider their patients' cultural backgrounds and how they might affect pain assessment and pain treatment. Unfortunately, health care systems may not understand or be sensitive to various cultural or religious backgrounds that may affect how patients express pain and how pain fits into patients' world views. The result can be poor communication, inadequate treatment, and increased pain and suffering. Pain-relief strategies that take into account an individual's cultural beliefs about pain have a much better chance of success.

Impact on Care

Cultural influences significantly affect communication between patient and doctor and impact the success of pain-management plans. For example, a patient who comes from a culture in which pain endurance is associated with strength and character may not be easily convinced to take prescribed pain medications. Health care providers who are aware of and who adjust to cultural differences among their patients are in a position to provide the most effective care to patients who are in pain.

Research indicates that patients from minority groups are less likely to receive the pain treatment they need than those from nonminority groups. Doctors may underestimate the severity of pain for these patients and may also be more likely to underestimate the severity of pain for female patients than for male patients.

Cultural differences may be related to socioeconomic status, education, access to health care, knowledge, attitudes toward doctors, patient behavior, and other factors. Cultural and language differences may also play a role because they can inhibit communication and understanding between patients and doctors (see chapter 3). These factors may result inadequate pain assessment, pain treatment, and follow-up care.

Because people from certain cultures may behave differently than others in the presence of pain, such as not complaining, health care providers may misjudge these patients' level of distress and therefore not treat their pain aggressively enough. Cultural influences may also cause patients to wait longer to seek out treatment for pain or to first visit traditional folk healers before seeing a doctor who practices western medical techniques, which may cause them to experience pain for longer than necessary.

Pain Control in Diverse Populations

According to the federal government (Agency for Healthcare Research and Quality), in general, minority group patients are likely to receive less adequate treatment for cancer pain than nonminorities. Research has shown that African Americans and Hispanics with pain due to metastatic cancer were three times more likely to receive inadequate pain treatment than nonminorities.

The barriers that impede pain control among minority groups may include:

- cultural differences
- language differences, causing health professionals to judge pain levels based on behavior rather than on a patient's description (often resulting in underestimation of pain)
- inaccurate and incomplete pain assessment
- less frequent follow-up care by medical professionals
- decreased access to appropriate medical care
- fear of addiction to opioid pain medications among patients
- reluctance of doctors to prescribe opioid pain medications
- economic disadvantages among minority populations
- inadequate insurance reimbursement for pain treatment

Do not assume that health care professionals are familiar with personal and cultural factors that have an impact on how you experience and cope with pain. Make sure the members of your health care team are aware of all of the factors—including cultural beliefs—that might affect your pain assessment and treatment decisions.

Some health care professionals may be more concerned about the potential for drug addiction in minority group patients who require opioids to control pain, although there is no evidence to suggest that minority groups are more likely to misuse pain-relief medications.

Cultural sensitivity is growing within the medical community as health care professionals become more aware of the importance of culture. Ideally, all members of your oncology team will be nonjudgmental, flexible, sensitive, and respectful of your cultural background and will identify your health-related cultural beliefs and practices. To bridge potential cultural gaps and ensure that you receive the best and most comprehensive care possible, discuss your needs and wishes with your medical team. With this knowledge, they can develop a pain-management plan that takes your cultural background into account. Staying silent about your beliefs can jeopardize the success of your treatment and can result in unnecessary pain and suffering. You will benefit if you discuss your own personal way of dealing with pain and how your cultural background may influence your behavior.

Treating Pain in the Person with Advanced Disease

"I still remember the day I received the call from Tom, my fifty-year-old brother, telling me he had a recurrence of melanoma. His disease had already spread to both lungs. We had many long talks in the days that followed. We spoke about the possibility of his death and he told me that his biggest fear was dying in pain. I reassured him that everything possible would be done to control his pain. He was more than my brother, he was a best friend."

—Susan, a cancer nurse

You may have heard the term palliative care. Palliative care is treatment that relieves suffering and improves the quality of a person's life by treating symptoms caused by the cancer or cancer treatment. Sometimes it may be referred to as supportive care. Palliative care is given to all patients throughout their cancer experience when they have symptoms caused by cancer or treatment. (See chapter 6.)

A person's cancer may at some point grow until it spreads to vital organs. If this occurs, it is called advanced cancer. As the cancer progresses and cancer treatment options become limited, palliative efforts become the major focus of care. As symptoms increase, more attention is needed to control them—especially as a person nears the end of life.

The goal of palliative care is to integrate comfort and pain relief with other medical care a patient may be receiving. Palliative care may be provided in varied environments, including medical centers and other acute-care hospitals, as well as in outpatient settings and by hospice teams for patients living at home or in assisted living facilities, nursing facilities, or inpatient hospices.

Palliative care includes not only medical treatments to relieve pain and other symptoms, but also emotional and spiritual support for patients and their loved ones.

Pain Relief at the End of Life

"Tom was started on a morphine drip with instructions that it be increased as needed. The next obstacle was with several members of the nursing staff. Being a nurse myself, this was a huge disappointment to me. Entire eight-hour shifts passed with my sister and I asking for the dose to be increased without success. One nurse actually asked me if I was 'trying to kill' my brother. His agony resulted not only from his untreated pain, but was intensified when the staff appeared not to believe his reports of pain. He was alert and expressed his feelings, but to little avail."

Pain relief improves the quality of one's life regardless of how serious the illness. But many patients do not receive adequate pain management at the end of life. Researchers continue to explore end-of-life pain management to try to discover how to better manage pain relief for people in pain at this stage.

Patients with a life-threatening disease such as cancer and their loved ones may have difficulty accepting the realization that their health care team can no longer cure their disease. Psychologists and counselors can provide both preparatory grief counseling for patients who are terminally ill and their loved ones, as well as bereavement counseling after the fact. Ideally, a person with advanced disease should talk with a mental health professional early in the course of treatment and throughout the course of the illness.

Treating Severe Pain in Advanced Stages of Cancer

Patients near the end of life may experience severe pain or other symptoms, including profound psychological distress. An estimated 70 to 90 percent of persons with advanced cancer experience pain—pain that can be eliminated, or at least reduced. Yet in many cases, and for a variety of reasons, some doctors are still reluctant to use all of the tools at their disposal to treat pain. In some cases, symptom management requires high doses of opioids and other types of pain-relief medications.

The goal of pain management for patients whose disease is advanced and who are in severe pain is to increase comfort while allowing them to remain in control of their life. This means that side effects are managed to ensure that patients experience as little pain as possible, yet remain alert enough to make decisions that they feel are important. However, high doses of opioids often result in a tradeoff between adequate pain control and decreased alertness, functional ability, and side effects of medication, such as confusion and hallucinations.

Sometimes, however, adequate pain management cannot be achieved without decreasing a patient's alertness. (See the *Palliative Sedation* section on page 180 for more information.) For example, high doses of opioids and sedatives may be needed to control pain. Side effects such as continual drowsiness and prolonged periods of sleep may be unavoidable in such cases. Any pain symptom that a patient finds intolerable should be taken very seriously and addressed aggressively with appropriate pain-management techniques. If the patient's regular doctor cannot find a solution, caregivers may decide to consult with a pain-management expert to find solutions.

Hospice Care

"The day came when Tom's melanoma spread to his central nervous system and his pain escalated dramatically. He was admitted to a hospital near my home and the 'nightmare' began. My first indication of a problem came with a call from Tom at 4:00 a.m. one morning. As I answered the phone, I heard him say, 'The pain is unbearable and they say there isn't anything else that

can be done.' I dressed and went to the hospital and from that day until his death, my sister and I took turns staying at his side. We served as his advocates in his struggle for pain relief that followed."

Hospice care focuses on providing humane and compassionate care for people in the last phases of an incurable disease so that they may live as fully and comfortably as possible surrounded by loved ones. It is appropriate when a patient can no longer benefit from attempts to cure cancer. Hospice care centers on treating the person, not the disease, and emphasizes quality of life rather than length of life.

Typically, hospice care involves a health care team of doctors, nurses, social workers, counselors, hospice-certified nursing assistants, religious and spiritual leaders, therapists, and volunteers—each offering support based on their own area of expertise. Together, they provide palliative care aimed at relieving symptoms, controlling pain, and providing supportive social, emotional, and spiritual care services. Care may take place at a patient's home, in a hospital, a nursing home, or an inpatient hospice unit.

Feel free to ask a doctor, nurse, or social worker to give you a list of local hospices. Hospice services are also listed in the yellow pages of the telephone book. There are agencies that can refer you to hospices in your community, such as the American Cancer Society, the Hospice Foundation of America, the National Association for Home Care & Hospice, and the National Hospice and Palliative Care Organization. See the *Resources* section at the end of this book for contact information.

Palliative Sedation

If severe pain persists after doctors with specialized expertise have explored all potential alternatives and the person with cancer is near the end of his or her life, the patient and family may consider palliative sedation in order to relieve suffering from severe unendurable symptoms that have not responded to treatment. Only a small percentage of patients have symptoms that might benefit from palliative sedation at the end of life.

The patient may have specified his or her wishes regarding palliative sedation in an advance directive (a legal document that tells the doctor and family what a person wants for future medical care, including whether to start or when to stop life-sustaining treatment), which may include detailed terms of care. The main objective of palliative sedation is to preserve a patient's comfort, which may require that the patient be asleep most of the day. A secondary effect of palliative sedation is that it may be hasten the end of life, because continuous sedation can impair the functioning of the heart and lungs.

Palliative sedation can involve one of several pharmacologic options. If a person is currently being treated with opioids, the opioid dose will usually be increased as a first step. But tolerance to opioids, and pain that is too intense can rule out this option. Sometimes a side effect of increasing the opioid dose may occur as well, such as severe muscle twitching. In these cases an adjuvant analgesic such as a neuroleptic, benzodiazepine, or barbiturate may be added.

Palliative sedation is different from euthanasia (see below). Palliative sedation is legally recognized and ethically justified in the care of the terminally ill. Psychological counseling with mental health professionals may aid loved ones under these difficult circumstances. If family members disagree on whether to take measures that could hasten the death of a patient yet will greatly ease pain, and the patient is no longer able to participate in medical decision-making, they should be guided by the patient's wishes, if they are known.

In contrast, euthanasia, which is illegal in the United States, is an action or omission that causes death with the purpose of ending suffering due to illness. Euthanasia occurs when a patient is terminally ill and voluntarily chooses to end his or her life in order to avoid prolonged suffering. While euthanasia is illegal, in 1994, Oregon voters approved the Death with Dignity Act, which allows a doctor to prescribe a lethal dose of medication requested by a competent, terminally ill person. The medication must be self-administered.

"From the beginning of his illness, taking control of the situation was very important to Tom. He took great satisfaction in making informed decisions and always having a plan. His plan was rewritten many, many times, and each new plan had fresh hope. His final plan was for a peaceful, pain-free death with dignity. I'm glad he's at peace."

Conclusion

Pain can decrease a person's ability to go about daily activities and enjoy life, but in most cases, pain from cancer and its treatments can be controlled. By developing an understanding of the issues related to the assessment and treatment of pain, how to talk about pain, and the wide variety of pain-relief options available, you and your health care team can work together to relieve cancer pain with minimal side effects.

The pain-prevention and pain-relief strategies in this book are aimed at improving your overall well-being and allowing you to take control of your life. Remember, everyone has the right to pain relief. Being informed about pain and its relief will help ensure that you receive the pain relief you deserve.

Appendixes

Appendix A: Cancer Pain Drug Information

NONOPIOIDS (for mild to moderate pain)

Drug Type	Generic Name and Trade Name	Action (Use)	Delivery Method
Antipyretic (fever-reducing) Analgesic	acetaminophen (Acephen, Actamin, Anacin-3, Apacet, Anesin, Dapa, Datril, Genapap, Genebs, Gentabs, Halenol, Liquiprin, Meda Cap, Panadol, Panex, Suppap, Tempra, Tenol, Ty Caps, Tylenol)	· relieves pain, decreases pain perception · reduces fever	· oral · rectal
Nonsteroidal anti-inflammatory drug (NSAID)	aspirin, acetylsalicyclic acid (acetylsalicyclic acid Bayer aspirin, Easprin, Ecotrin, Empirin)	· decreases pain perception · reduces inflammation · reduces fever · relieves pain	· oral · rectal
NSAID	ibuprofen (Advil, Genpril, Haltran, Ibuprin, Midol 200, Nuprin, Rufen)	· decreases pain perception · reduces inflammation · reduces fever · relieves pain	· oral
NSAID	salsalate (Disalcid, Salsalate, Salflex)	· decreases pain perception · reduces inflammation · reduces fever	· oral
NSAID	choline magnesium trisalicylate (Trilisate)	· decreases pain perception · reduces inflammation · reduces fever	· oral
NSAID	celecoxib (Celebrex)	· decreases pain perception · reduces inflammation	· oral

Side Effects

MORE COMMON:	LESS COMMON:
· None	· possible liver damage in those who consume three or more alcoholic drinks a day, or in those with liver or kidney disease · few side effects when taken as directed

MORE COMMON:		LESS COMMON:	
· increased bleeding time · heartburn	· increased bruising · sweating	· bleeding in gastrointestinal tract · flushing	· ringing in the ears · hearing loss · dizziness

MORE COMMON:		LESS COMMON:	
· dizziness · heartburn	· nausea · drowsiness	· vomiting · constipation · loss of appetite · diarrhea · sores in mouth or on lips · bloating · abdominal pain · bleeding from the gastrointestinal tract	· headache · nervousness · fatigue · anxiety · confusion · depression · mood swings · peptic ulcers

MORE COMMON:	LESS COMMON:	
· dizziness	· nausea · heartburn · loss of appetite · increased risk of peptic ulcer · ringing in the ears	· vomiting · diarrhea · confusion · lethargy · headache · sweating

MORE COMMON:	LESS COMMON:	
· None	· flushing · dizziness	· decreased hearing · ringing in the ears

MORE COMMON:		LESS COMMON:	
· abdominal pain · diarrhea · indigestion · gas · nausea · back pain · edema in the extremities	· dizziness · headache · inability to sleep · sore throat · runny nose · rash	· constipation · difficulty swallowing · gastroenteritis · acid reflux · vomiting · chest pain · increased blood pressure · allergic reaction · rash	· flu-like symptoms · leg cramps · migraine · ringing in the ears · change in liver and kidney function · problems with blood clotting · difficulty with urination

NONOPIOIDS (for mild to moderate pain)

Drug Type	Generic Name and Trade Name	Action (Use)	Delivery Method
NSAID	diclofenac (Voltaren)	· decreases pain perception · reduces inflammation	· oral
NSAID	diflunisal (Dolobid)	· decreases pain perception · reduces inflammation	· oral
NSAID	fenoprofen (Nalfon)	· decreases pain perception · reduces inflammation	· oral
NSAID	ketoprofen (Orudis)	· decreases pain perception · reduces inflammation	· oral

MORE COMMON:
- nausea
- vomiting
- heartburn
- gastrointestinal bleeding
- headache
- dizziness
- changes in liver function
- diarrhea
- constipation
- rash
- itching
- ringing in the ears

LESS COMMON:
- swelling of lips and tongue
- allergic reaction
- increased blood pressure
- congestive heart failure
- vomiting
- yellow skin
- anemia
- inability to sleep
- drowsiness
- depression
- anxiety
- double or blurred vision
- irritability
- nose bleed
- asthma
- chest pain
- bruising
- tingling
- frequent urination

MORE COMMON:
- abdominal pain
- constipation
- diarrhea
- dizziness
- fatigue
- headache
- inability to sleep
- indigestion
- nausea
- rash
- ringing in ears
- sleepiness
- vomiting

LESS COMMON:
- gastrointestinal bleeding
- anemia
- blurred vision
- confusion
- depression
- disorientation
- dry mouth and nose
- fluid retention
- flushing
- changes in liver function
- hives
- inflammation of lips and tongue
- itching
- changes in kidney function
- light-headedness
- loss of appetite
- nervousness
- gastric ulcer
- tingling in the extremities
- protein or blood in urine, difficulty urinating

MORE COMMON:
- indigestion
- nausea
- constipation
- vomiting
- abdominal pain
- diarrhea
- headache
- drowsiness
- dizziness
- sweating
- ringing in the ears
- blurred vision
- palpitations
- nervousness
- tingling
- swelling in the extremities
- shortness of breath
- fatigue

LESS COMMON:
- gastritis
- peptic ulcer with and without perforation
- gastrointestinal bleeding
- loss of appetite
- gas
- dry mouth
- change in liver function
- change in kidney function
- allergic reaction
- bruising

MORE COMMON:
- indigestion
- nausea
- vomiting
- diarrhea
- constipation
- headache
- dizziness
- drowsiness
- depression
- anxiety
- ringing in the ears
- rash
- visual disturbances
- change in renal function

LESS COMMON:
- gastrointestinal bleeding
- increased blood pressure and heart rate
- change in liver function
- bleeding problems
- muscle pain
- confusion
- migraine
- shortness of breath
- sweating
- rash

NONOPIOIDS (for mild to moderate pain)

Drug Type	Generic Name and Trade Name	Action (Use)	Delivery Method
NSAID	piroxicam (Feldene)	· decreases pain perception · reduces inflammation · reduces fever	· oral
NSAID	indomethacin (Indocin)	· decreases pain perception · reduces inflammation · reduces fever	· oral
NSAID	naproxen (Naprosyn)	· decreases pain perception · reduces inflammation	· oral
NSAID	rofecoxib (Vioxx)	· decreases pain perception · reduces inflammation	· oral
NSAID	ketorolac tromethamine (Toradol)	· decreases pain perception · reduces inflammation · reduces fever · only NSAID that can be given by injection	· IV · oral · IM*

*IM route is to be avoided if at all possible

MORE COMMON:
- swelling of the extremities
- nausea
- heartburn
- gastric ulcers
- gastointestinal bleeding
- diarrhea
- ringing in the ears
- drowsiness
- nervousness
- dry mouth
- abnormal kidney function

LESS COMMON:
- changes in liver function
- allergic reaction
- rash
- itching
- depression
- increased blood sugar
- anemia
- dizziness
- headache
- asthma
- increased blood pressure

MORE COMMON:
- headache
- vomiting
- ringing in ears (tinnitus)
- tremors
- sleeplessness

LESS COMMON:
- dizziness
- depression
- fatigue
- numbness and tingling in hands and/or feet
- nausea
- loss of appetite
- heartburn, indigestion, epigastric pain
- bleeding from gastrointestinal tract

MORE COMMON:
- constipation
- heartburn
- abdominal pain
- nausea
- indigestion
- diarrhea
- mouth sores
- headache
- dizziness
- drowsiness
- itching
- rash
- sweating
- ringing in the ears
- swelling of the extremities
- shortness of breath

LESS COMMON:
- abnormal liver function
- gastrointestinal bleeding and/or perforation
- vomiting
- yellowing of skin
- alteration in kidney function
- low platelet count
- low white blood cell count
- depression
- difficulty sleeping
- itching
- hearing changes
- allergic reaction

MORE COMMON:
- abdominal pain
- fatigue
- dizziness
- flu-like symptoms
- swelling in legs
- upper respiratory infection
- increased blood pressure
- indigestion
- heartburn
- nausea
- sinusitis
- back pain
- headache
- bronchitis
- urinary tract infection

LESS COMMON:
- dry mouth
- inflammation of the esophagus
- gas
- acid reflux
- allergic reaction
- weight gain
- increased blood cholesterol
- muscle pain
- depression
- anxiety
- asthma
- rash
- difficulty urinating

MORE COMMON:
- heartburn
- dizziness
- drowsiness
- lightheadedness

LESS COMMON:
- nausea
- vomiting
- loss of appetite
- diarrhea
- constipation
- sores in mouth or on lips
- bloating
- abdominal pain
- peptic ulcers
- bleeding from gastrointestinal tract
- headache
- nervousness
- fatigue
- anxiety
- confusion
- depression
- mood swings

OPIOIDS (for moderate to severe pain)

Drug Type	Generic Name and Trade Name	Action (Use)	Delivery Method
Opioid	codeine—when combined with acetaminophen (Phenaphen with codeine, Tylenol with codeine, Tylenol 3) codeine—when combined with aspirin (Empirin with codeine, Soma Compound with codeine, Fiorinal with codeine)	· relieves mild to moderate pain · alters the perception of pain	· IV · oral · IM*
Opioid	fentanyl citrate (Actiq)	· relieves moderate to severe pain · alters the perception of pain · used for breakthrough pain or before procedures	· transmucosal: lozenge on a stick/handle, to be placed between cheek and lower gum
Opioid	fentanyl transdermal system (Duragesic)	· relieves moderate to severe pain · alters the perception of pain	· skin patch
Opioid	hydromorphone (Dilaudid)	· relieves moderate to severe pain · is similar to morphine · alters the perception of pain	· IV · oral · IM*
Opioid	levorphanol tartrate (Levo-Dromoran)	· relieves moderate to severe pain · similar to morphine · alters the perception of pain	· IV · SQ · oral

*IM route is to be avoided if at all possible

Side Effects

MORE COMMON:
- nausea
- constipation
- drowsiness
- sedation
- mood changes
- dizziness
- dry mouth

LESS COMMON:
- euphoria
- depression
- mental clouding
- vomiting
- dizziness when changing position
- flushing
- itching
- sweating
- decreased heart rate
- difficulty urinating

MORE COMMON:
- sleepiness
- dizziness
- headache
- fever
- fatigue
- constipation

LESS COMMON:
- difficulty breathing
- cough
- sore throat
- sedation
- anxiety
- confusion
- depression
- difficulty sleeping
- muscle aches
- itching
- rash
- sweating
- nausea
- vomiting
- loss of appetite
- heartburn

MORE COMMON:
- sleepiness
- dizziness
- constipation
- nausea

LESS COMMON:
- difficulty breathing
- decreased breathing rate
- confusion
- depression
- nervousness
- tremors
- lack of coordination
- euphoria
- difficulty speaking
- vomiting
- chest pain
- decreased blood pressure when changing position
- sweating
- difficulty urinating
- rash
- itching

MORE COMMON:
- constipation
- drowsiness
- sedation
- dizziness
- nausea
- dry mouth

LESS COMMON:
- mood changes
- euphoria
- mental clouding
- decreased breathing rate
- vomiting
- delayed digestion
- decreased blood pressure when changing position
- decreased heart rate

MORE COMMON:
- constipation
- drowsiness
- sedation
- nausea
- dry mouth

LESS COMMON:
- changes in mood
- euphoria
- depression
- mental clouding
- decreased rate of breathing
- vomiting
- delayed digestion
- decreased blood pressure when changing position
- decreased heart rate

OPIOIDS (for moderate to severe pain)

Drug Type	Generic Name and Trade Name	Action (Use)	Delivery Method
Opioid	meperidine hydrochloride (Demerol); merperidine with promethazine (Mepergan Fortis)	· relieves moderate to severe pain · alters the perception of pain · not an effective choice for chronic cancer pain	· IV · oral · SQ · IM*
Opioid	methadone (Dolophine)	· relieves moderate to severe pain · alters the perception of pain	· SQ · oral · IM*
Opioid	morphine (Astramorph, Duramorph, Infumorph, Kadian, Morphine Sulfate Sustained Release, MS Contin, MSIR, Oramorph, Roxanol)	· relieves moderate to severe pain · alters the perception of pain	· IV · SQ · by infusion · rectal · into spinal canal
Opioid	oxycodone (OxyContin, Roxicodone); oxycodone with aspirin (Percodan, Endodan, Roxiprin); oxycodone with acetaminophen (Percocet)	· relieves moderate to severe pain · alters the perception of pain	· oral

*IM route is to be avoided if at all possible

Side Effects

MORE COMMON:
- constipation
- drowsiness
- sedation
- nausea
- vomiting
- dizziness
- dry mouth

LESS COMMON:
- changes in mood
- euphoria
- mental clouding
- decreased breathing rate
- decreased blood pressure when changing position
- delayed digestion
- decreased heart rate

MORE COMMON:
- constipation
- drowsiness
- sedation
- nausea
- dizziness
- dry mouth

LESS COMMON:
- vomiting
- changes in mood
- euphoria
- depression
- mental clouding
- decreased breathing rate
- decreased blood pressure when changing position
- delayed digestion
- decreased heart rate

MORE COMMON:
- constipation
- drowsiness
- sedation
- nausea
- dizziness
- dry mouth

LESS COMMON:
- vomiting
- changes in mood
- euphoria
- depression
- mental clouding
- decreased breathing rate
- decreased blood pressure when changing position
- delayed digestion
- decreased heart rate

MORE COMMON:
- constipation
- drowsiness
- sedation
- nausea
- dizziness
- dry mouth

LESS COMMON:
- vomiting
- changes in mood
- euphoria
- depression
- mental clouding
- decreased breathing rate
- decreased blood pressure when changing position
- delayed digestion
- decreased heart rate

ADJUVANT ANALGESICS
(antianxiety drugs, anticonvulsants, antidepressants, steroids)

Drug Type	Generic Name and Trade Name	Action (Use)	Delivery Method
Antianxiety	buspirone hydrochloride (Buspar)	· action not known, but it affects the neurotransmitters in the brain that bring about the feeling of anxiety	· oral
Antianxiety	alprazolam (Xanax)	· reduces anxiety · muscle relaxant · anticonvulsant effects	· oral
Antianxiety	clonazepam (Klonopin)	· manages anxiety, panic attacks, seizures, involuntary movements	· oral
Antianxiety	diazepam (Valium)	· reduces anxiety · causes muscle relaxation · prevents seizures	· IV · oral · IM*
Antianxiety	lorazepam (Ativan)	· reduces anxiety · causes muscle relaxation · prevents seizures · decreases chance of nausea and vomiting following chemotherapy · causes amnesia	· IV · oral · SQ · IM*
Antianxiety	oxazepam (Serax)	· reduces anxiety · relaxes muscles · prevents seizures	· oral
Antinausea Antivomiting Antianxiety	haloperidol (Haldol)	· prevents nausea and vomiting resulting from chemotherapy · decreases agitation	· oral · IM*

*IM route is to be avoided if at all possible

Side Effects

MORE COMMON:		LESS COMMON:	
· None		· dizziness	· headache
		· drowsiness	

MORE COMMON:		LESS COMMON:	
· dry mouth	· decreased mental alertness	· nausea	· change in body weight
		· vomiting	
The following side effects occur when first starting the drug:			
· drowsiness	· weakness		
· fatigue	· confusion		
· lethargy	· headache		

MORE COMMON:		LESS COMMON:	
· drowsiness		· decrease in blood pressure when changing position	· decreased mental alertness
			· dizziness

MORE COMMON:		LESS COMMON:	
The following side effects occur when first starting the drug:		· feeling "hung over" the next day	· decreased mental alertness
· drowsiness	· confusion	· decreased coordination	· decreased in blood pressure
· feeling tired	· headache		· decreased heart rate

MORE COMMON:		LESS COMMON:	
The following side effects occur when first starting the drug:		· nausea	· decreased mental alertness
· drowsiness	· weakness	· dry mouth	· change in heart rate
· fatigue	· headache	· constipation	· change in blood pressure
· confusion		· lack of coordination	

MORE COMMON:		LESS COMMON:	
· drowsiness	· dry mouth	· nausea	· lack of coordination
· fatigue	· constipation	· vomiting	· decreased mental alertness
· weakness		· change in weight	

MORE COMMON:		LESS COMMON:	
· feeling sedated	· sleepiness	· decreased breathing rate	· decrease in blood pressure when changing position
		· increased heart rate	

ADJUVANT ANALGESICS
(antianxiety drugs, anticonvulsants, antidepressants, steroids)

Drug Type	Generic Name and Trade Name	Action (Use)	Delivery Method
Anticonvulsant	gabapentin (Neurontin)	· helpful in treating neuropathic pain	· oral
Antidepressant	doxepin hydrochloride (Sinequan)	· decreases or stops the feeling of depression	· oral
Antidepressant	nefazodone hydrochloride (Serzone)	· prevents or relieves depression	· oral
Antidepressant	trazodone hydrochloride (Desyrel, Trialodine)	· decreases the feeling of depression	· oral
Antidepressant	venlafaxine hydrochloride (Effexor)	· prevents or relieves the feeling of depression	· oral
Antidepressant: Selective Serotonin Reuptake Inhibitor (SSRI)	fluoxetine hydrochloride (Prozac)	· decreases the feeling of depression	· oral
Antidepressant: Selective Serotonin Reuptake Inhibitor (SSRI)	paroxetine hydrochloride (Paxil)	· decreases the feeling of depression	· oral

Side Effects

MORE COMMON:
- sleepiness
- dizziness
- fatigue

LESS COMMON:
- difficulty walking
- tremors
- nervousness
- difficulty speaking
- amnesia
- depression
- decreased muscle coordination
- headache
- confusion
- mood swings
- numbness in hands and/or feet
- decreased reflexes
- irritability
- heartburn
- nausea
- vomiting
- rash
- hair thinning

MORE COMMON:
- drowsiness

LESS COMMON:
- dry mouth
- decreased appetite
- indigestion
- changes in taste including metallic taste of foods
- urinary retention

MORE COMMON:
- dizziness
- drowsiness
- difficulty sleeping
- dry mouth
- nausea
- constipation
- headache
- feeling "blah"

LESS COMMON:
- lightheadedness
- heartburn

MORE COMMON:
- drowsiness
- dizziness
- lightheadedness
- decrease in blood pressure when changing from a lying or sitting position to standing

LESS COMMON:
- fatigue
- nightmares
- confusion
- anger
- excitement
- decreased mental concentration
- disorientation
- nervousness
- difficulty remembering

MORE COMMON:
- migraine headache
- dizziness when standing up
- tightness in the jaw
- nausea

LESS COMMON:
- loss of appetite
- constipation
- problem in sexual function
- feeling "blah"
- neck pain
- hangover-like effect
- bone pain
- black and blue spots on the skin
- problems urinating

MORE COMMON:
- headache

LESS COMMON:
- difficulty speaking
- anxiety
- decreased ability to concentrate
- tremor
- dizziness
- nausea
- loss of appetite
- weight loss in underweight individuals
- muscle or bone pain

MORE COMMON:
- sweating

LESS COMMON:
- sleepiness
- dizziness
- difficulty sleeping
- tremors
- nervousness
- feeling "blah"
- nausea
- decreased appetite
- decreased sexual ability

ADJUVANT ANALGESICS
(antianxiety drugs, anticonvulsants, antidepressants, steroids)

Drug Type	Generic Name and Trade Name	Action (Use)	Delivery Method
Antidepressant: Tricyclic	amitriptyline hydrochloride (Elavil)	· prevents and relieves depression · reduces peripheral nerve pain	· oral
Antidepressant: Tricyclic	desipramine hydrochloride (Norpramin, Pertofrane)	· prevents or relieves depression · reduces pain related to peripheral neuropathy	· oral
Antidepressant: Tricyclic	imipramine pamoate (Tofranil-PM)	· decreases or stops the feeling of depression · promotes sleep · treats hiccups	· oral · IM*
Antidepressant: Tricyclic	nortriptyline hydrochloride (Aventyl, Pamelor)	· decreases the feeling of depression · increases pain relief from narcotic drugs	· oral
Corticosteroid	prednisone (Apo-prednisone, Deltasone, Orasone, Prednisone)	· decreases inflammation	· oral
Corticosteroid	dexamethasone (Decadron)	· relieves nausea associated with chemotherapy · reduces swelling of the brain	· IV · oral

*IM route is to be avoided if at all possible

MORE COMMON:
- drowsiness
- dizziness
- weakness
- lethargy
- fatigue
- dry mouth

LESS COMMON:
- confusion (especially in the elderly)
- disorientation
- hallucinations
- decreased blood pressure when changing position
- increased heart rate
- increased blood pressure
- loss of appetite
- nausea
- vomiting
- diarrhea
- urinary retention

MORE COMMON:
- drowsiness
- dizziness
- weakness
- fatigue
- dry mouth

LESS COMMON:
- confusion (especially in the elderly)
- disorientation
- hallucinations
- increased heart rate
- decrease in blood pressure when changing position
- loss of appetite
- urinary retention

MORE COMMON:
- drowsiness
- dizziness
- weakness
- fatigue

LESS COMMON:
- confusion
- disorientation
- change in blood pressure when changing position
- increased heart rate
- dry mouth
- decreased appetite
- nausea
- urinary retention

MORE COMMON:
- drowsiness
- fatigue
- dizziness
- dry mouth
- vomiting
- diarrhea
- abdominal cramping

LESS COMMON:
- confusion
- disorientation
- nausea
- changes in appetite
- urinary retention

MORE COMMON:
- delayed wound healing
- mood changes
- depression
- increased blood sugar
- increased appetite with weight gain
- bruising of the skin
- sleep disturbance
- increased risk of infection
- sodium and fluid retention with swelling in ankles, increased blood pressure, and congestive heart failure

LESS COMMON:
- decreased blood potassium level (symptoms are loss of appetite, muscle twitching, increased thirst, increased urination)
- weakness
- fracture of weak bones
- sweating
- fungal infections (white patches in mouth, vagina)
- diarrhea
- nausea
- headache
- increased heart rate
- loss of calcium from bones

MORE COMMON:
- increased appetite
- irritation of stomach
- euphoria
- difficulty sleeping
- mood changes
- flushing
- increased blood sugar
- decreased blood potassium level

LESS COMMON:
- depression
- headache
- sweating
- increased blood pressure

Appendix B: Guidelines for Pain Management

In recent years, more attention has focused on the issue of cancer pain. Professional nurse, physician, and health care organizations have developed standards for education, training, and patient care to ensure that people with cancer pain are receiving appropriate care. Below are some of the current organizations that have developed guidelines and standards related to cancer pain. These guidelines help guide physicians, health care teams, and health care facilities in making appropriate decisions about the treatment of cancer pain.

Joint Commission on the Accreditation of Healthcare Organizations

The Joint Commission on the Accreditation of Healthcare Organizations (JCAHO) is responsible for accrediting hospitals, ambulatory care centers, some long-term care centers, and other facilities where people go for medical treatment. The Commission has issued pain-management guidelines for health care facilities that require health professionals to document a patient's level of pain. While in the hospital, patients are asked to rate their pain at all stages of treatment using a numeric scale so it can be tracked and attended to regularly. Hospitals are rated on their compliance with these guidelines.

American Pain Society

The 2003 version of the *Guideline for the Management of Cancer Pain in Adults and Children* is a comprehensive guideline for health care professionals that provides an update to previous guidelines from the Agency for Healthcare Research.

National Comprehensive Cancer Network

The National Comprehensive Cancer Network (NCCN) is a non-profit organization that is an alliance of 19 cancer centers across the country. Physicians and other health care professionals have developed clinical practice guidelines that serve as the practice standard for cancer treatment. Each year a panel of scientific experts updates clinical guidelines, based on advances in medical science and cancer treatment. The American Cancer Society has partnered with NCCN to translate the professional guidelines into a patient-friendly resource. These guidelines offer easy-to-understand information for patients and family members about treatment options (see *Resources*).

The *Cancer Pain Treatment Guidelines for Patients* that follow—which are based on professional guidelines—will help you understand your options for pain management. The "decision trees" show step-by-step treatment options for pain control. With this information, you'll be better prepared to discuss your choices with your doctor.

Cancer Pain Treatment Guidelines for Patients

Decision Trees

The "decision trees," or algorithms, on the following pages represent decisions about treatment of cancer pain based on how bad the pain is. Each tree shows step-by-step how you and your doctor can make treatment choices.

Keep in mind, this information is not meant to be used without the expertise of your own doctor who is familiar with your situation, medical history, and personal preferences.

The NCCN guidelines are updated as new significant data become available. For the most recent information on these guidelines or on cancer in general, contact the American Cancer Society (800-ACS-2345; http://www.cancer.org) or the National Comprehensive Cancer Network (888-909-NCCN; http://www.nccn.org).

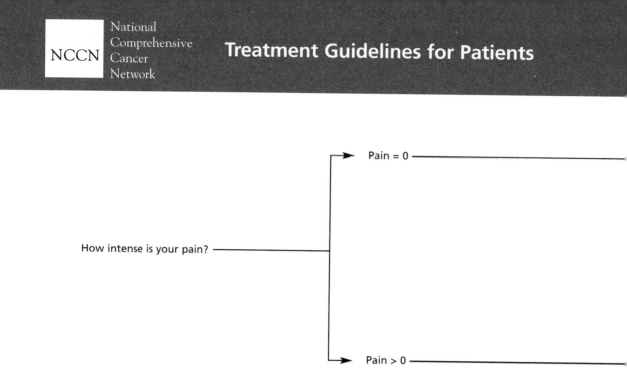

Pain = 0

How intense is your pain?

Pain > 0

Keep in mind, this information is not meant to be used without the expertise of your own physician who is familiar with your situation, medical history, and personal preferences.

Assessing the Patient's Pain (Does the patient have pain?)

Since all patients can have cancer pain but not all patients do, the first step in making a decision about treatment is to find out if the patient is having pain. The patient is asked to rate their pain using a visual rating scale of 1-10. A score of 0 indicates that no pain is present and a rating of 10 indicates the pain is the worst it can be. If the patient has no pain, he or she will be asked about it on each subsequent visit to the doctor. If the patient is in pain, the doctor will do a thorough assessment, or evaluation, so appropriate treatment can be planned.

The immediate goal of the first pain assessment is to find out if the pain is present because of a medical emergency. If one is present, it will require immediate treatment. Because tumors can invade bone, nerves, and tissue, there are several cancer pain emergencies that must be treated quickly. These include:

Decision Tree for the Assessment of Cancer-Related Pain

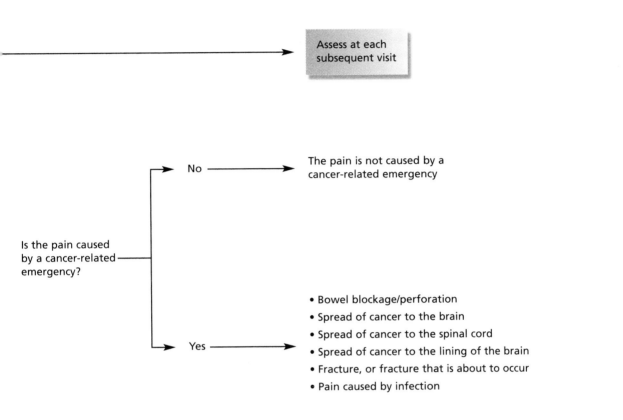

Assess at each subsequent visit

Is the pain caused by a cancer-related emergency?

No → The pain is not caused by a cancer-related emergency

Yes →
- Bowel blockage/perforation
- Spread of cancer to the brain
- Spread of cancer to the spinal cord
- Spread of cancer to the lining of the brain
- Fracture, or fracture that is about to occur
- Pain caused by infection

- a fracture (break in a bone) or near fracture of a bone that is able to carry weight, such as a vertebra in the back or the hip bone;

- a bowel blockage or perforation (hole in the wall of the bowel) caused by tumor growth;

- metastasis, or spread of the cancer to the brain, spinal cord, or the lining of the brain; and

- pain caused by an infection in just one part of the body, or one that involves the entire body (septicemia).

The patient will be asked several questions about their pain. The patient's completed numerical rating scale will help the doctor understand how intense, or bad, the pain is.

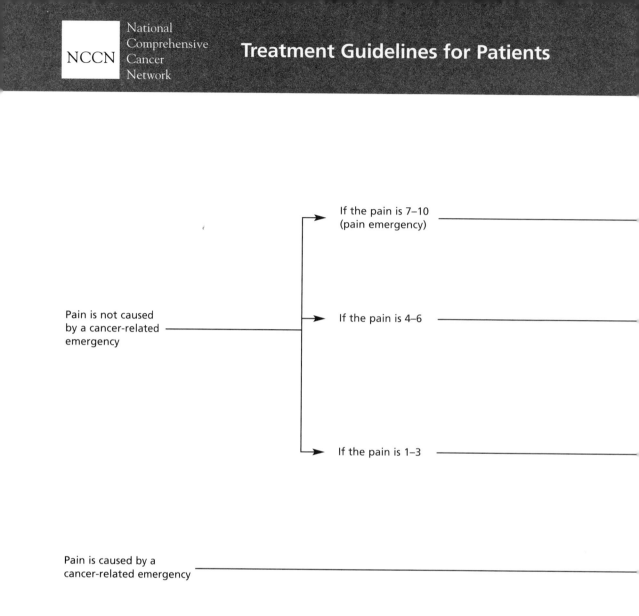

Pain is not caused by a cancer-related emergency

If the pain is 7–10 (pain emergency) _____

If the pain is 4–6 _____

If the pain is 1–3 _____

Pain is caused by a cancer-related emergency _____

Keep in mind, this information is not meant to be used without the expertise of your own physician who is familiar with your situation, medical history, and personal preferences.

Initial Treatment

Once the assessment is completed, the pain treatment is planned. Treatment options will be discussed with the patient. If it is a pain emergency, the cause of the pain will be treated.

If no emergency situation is present, and the patient's pain is greater than 7 on the visual pain scale, the patient will be given a short-acting opioid and the dose will be increased rapidly. A bowel program will be started to

Decision Tree for the Initial Treatment of Cancer-Related Pain

Initial Treatment

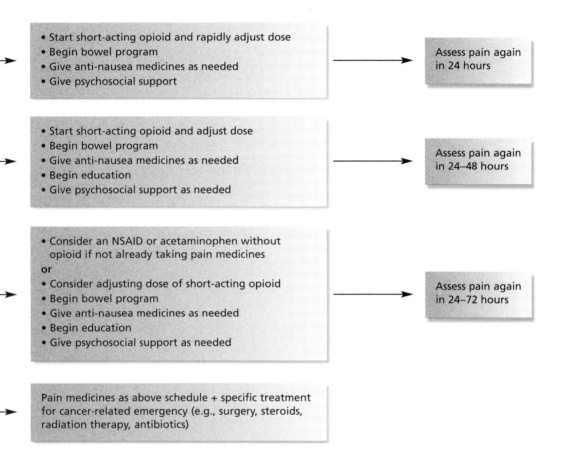

• Start short-acting opioid and rapidly adjust dose
• Begin bowel program
• Give anti-nausea medicines as needed
• Give psychosocial support

→ Assess pain again in 24 hours

• Start short-acting opioid and adjust dose
• Begin bowel program
• Give anti-nausea medicines as needed
• Begin education
• Give psychosocial support as needed

→ Assess pain again in 24–48 hours

• Consider an NSAID or acetaminophen without opioid if not already taking pain medicines
or
• Consider adjusting dose of short-acting opioid
• Begin bowel program
• Give anti-nausea medicines as needed
• Begin education
• Give psychosocial support as needed

→ Assess pain again in 24–72 hours

Pain medicines as above schedule + specific treatment for cancer-related emergency (e.g., surgery, steroids, radiation therapy, antibiotics)

lower the chances of constipation. A medicine may be given to prevent nausea and vomiting, a side effect from the opioid. During this time the patient will need the support of the cancer care team, family, and friends. In about 24 hours the pain will be re-evaluated using the pain rating scale.

If the pain is rated from 4–6, a short-acting opioid will be given with dose titrated, or adjusted (either increased or decreased) until the pain is relieved. The bowel preparation and "as needed" anti-nausea medicines will be started. Pain will be reassessed, or re-evaluated, in about 24–48 hours by the doctor or nurse.

If the pain is rated from 1–3, an NSAID or a short-acting opioid is an option. A bowel regimen will be started and anti-nausea medicines will be given "as needed." An education program should be started to establish a common language for talking about pain with the health care team. One goal of the education program is to understand why patients do not always get effective pain control and to make sure patients have the information they need to follow the prescribed plan. Beliefs that create the greatest problems for patients in taking their pain

NOTES

medicines are fear of addiction, concerns about side effects, concerns about tolerance, and the need to be stoic. Patients also should know what medicines they should stop taking and when to call the doctor.

Pain that is caused by a cancer-related emergency will be treated with analgesics, or pain medicines, according to the above treatment plan. Specific treatment will also be given for the emergency (for example, surgery, radiation therapy, antibiotics, or steroids).

In about 24–72 hours after the pain treatment is begun, the patient will complete another visual pain rating. Further changes in the pain treatment will be made based on how well the patient's pain is being controlled with the pain medicine.

NOTES

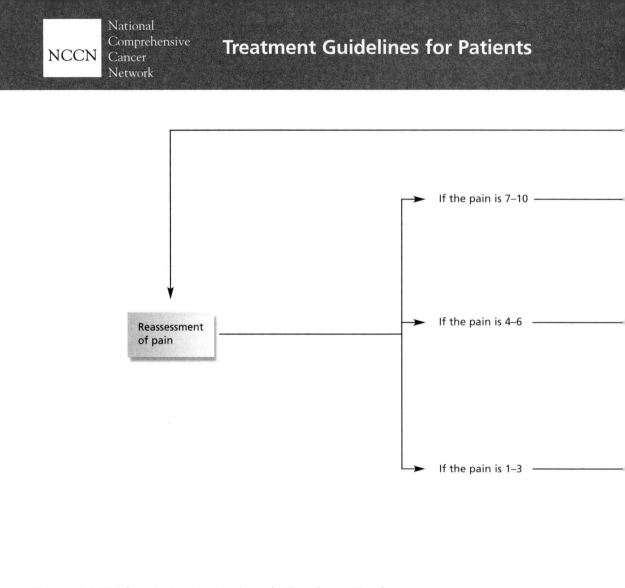

If the pain is 7–10 ——————

Reassessment of pain

If the pain is 4–6 ——————

If the pain is 1–3 ——————

Keep in mind, this information is not meant to be used without the expertise of your own physician who is familiar with your situation, medical history, and personal preferences.

Subsequent Treatment

A score of 7–10 means that the pain is not better or it has gotten worse. Since the goal of pain treatment is to reach a lower score on the pain scale, the doctor will reconsider the original cause of pain. This means that the doctor will look once again at the medical history and

consider if the original cause of pain is still causing the current pain.

Next, the patient's pain medicine dose will be adjusted. For example, more of the medicine may be given or a different medicine may be given. Additional treatments for specific types of pain may be added to the current pain

Decision Tree for the Subsequent Treatment of Cancer-Related Pain

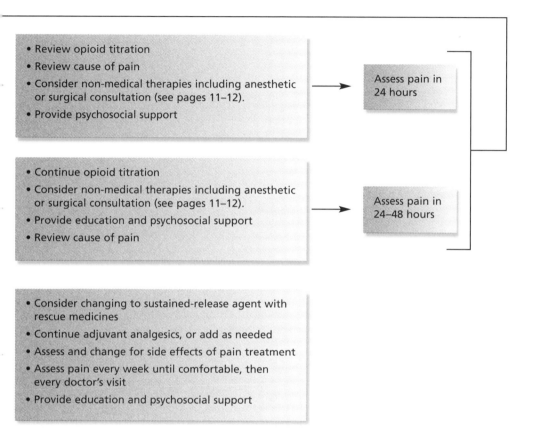

- Review opioid titration
- Review cause of pain
- Consider non-medical therapies including anesthetic or surgical consultation (see pages 11–12).
- Provide psychosocial support

Assess pain in 24 hours

- Continue opioid titration
- Consider non-medical therapies including anesthetic or surgical consultation (see pages 11–12).
- Provide education and psychosocial support
- Review cause of pain

Assess pain in 24–48 hours

- Consider changing to sustained-release agent with rescue medicines
- Continue adjuvant analgesics, or add as needed
- Assess and change for side effects of pain treatment
- Assess pain every week until comfortable, then every doctor's visit
- Provide education and psychosocial support

medicines. For example, NSAIDs might be added with bone pain or pain with inflammation. Antidepressants might be added for burning neuropathic pain. Non-medical therapies will also be considered. The pain will be re-evaluated in about 24 hours.

If the patient's pain score is 4–6, the doctor will continue to adjust the medicine dose. Other treatments (as mentioned above) may also be added. After changes have been made in the pain treatment plan, the patient's pain will be assessed in about 24–48 hours to see if it is any better.

If the pain is rated 3 or less, the pain medicine may be switched to a sustained-released oral medicine, which means the patient can take the medicine less often. Medicine will be given if the patient has breakthrough pain. Other medicines that have been added to the pain treatment plan will be continued if they are still needed for the pain. Education and support will be continued as needed. The side effects of pain medicines will be considered and medicines will be changed if needed to reduce side effects. Pain will be assessed every week until the patient is comfortable, then with every visit to the doctor.

NOTES

The goal of pain treatment is to continue to reduce the amount of pain the patient has to a level less than 4. Pain is assessed after each change in treatment. Patient and family education and psychosocial support, important components of cancer pain treatment, are continued throughout treatment. After each pain assessment, pain treatment will be adjusted based on the intensity of the pain using the pain scale.

NOTES

Resources

American Cancer Society

The American Cancer Society is the nationwide community-based volunteer health organization dedicated to eliminating cancer as a major health problem by preventing cancer, saving lives and diminishing suffering from cancer, through research, education, advocacy, and service.

Additional materials related to pain available from the Society include:

- *Detailed Guide: Cancer Pain*
- *Pain Control: A Guide for People with Cancer and Their Families*
- *Breakthrough Cancer Pain: Questions and Answers*
- *NCCN Cancer Pain Treatment Guidelines for Patients*

For more information about cancer and cancer pain, educational materials (Spanish materials are available), patient programs, and services within your community, contact us:

Toll-free: 800-ACS-2345 (800-227-2345; 24-hour hotline)

Web site: http://www.cancer.org

About the Resources

Listings in this section represent organizations that operate on a national level and provide some type of service or resource to consumers related to cancer, cancer research, or public health. This list is designed to offer a starting point for seeking information, support, and needed resources. Most of the organizations listed here can be contacted via phone, fax, or e-mail, and some through their Web sites. Many of the Web sites provide much of the same information that is available by postal mail. Some organizations are solely Web-based and will require Internet access. Keep in mind that new Web sites appear daily while old ones expand, move, or disappear entirely. Some of the Web sites or content outlined below may change. Often, a simple Internet search will point to the new Web site for a given organization. The American Cancer Society Web site provides links to outside sources of cancer information as well (http://www.cancer.org; click on Cancer Resource Center).

There is a vast amount of information on the Internet. This information can be very valuable to the general public in making decisions about their health. However, since any group or individual can publish on the Internet, it is important to consider the credentials and reputation of the organization providing information. Internet information should not be a substitute for medical advice.

The American Cancer Society does not necessarily endorse the agencies, organizations, corporations, and publications represented in this resource guide. This guide is provided for assistance in obtaining information only.

Pain and Cancer Information

The organizations listed below provide information about pain and cancer. Most of the Web sites provided are searchable under the topic of pain and some have special sections devoted exclusively to pain and related issues.

American Alliance of Cancer Pain Initiatives (AACPI)
Resource Center
1300 University Avenue, Room 4720
Madison, WI 53706
Phone: 608-265-4013
Fax: 608-265-4014
Web site: http://wiscinfo.doit.wisc.edu/trc/

This organization promotes cancer pain relief by supporting the growth, development, and advocacy of state cancer pain initiatives. The resource center offers a variety of education resources about pain management, such as patient education booklets, videos, information about analgesic patient assistance programs, and e-mail newsletters.

American Pain Foundation
201 N. Charles Street, Suite 710
Baltimore, MD 21201-4111
Toll-Free: 888-615-PAIN (888-615-7246; automated request line)
Fax: 410-385-1832
Web site: http://www.painfoundation.org

This independent nonprofit organization serves people with pain through information, education, and advocacy. Their Web site includes an online support group program and educational materials, including the *Pain Action Guide*, *Pain Care Bill of Rights* (in English and Spanish) and the *Pain Community Newsletter*. Call for materials and for help finding trained specialists and peer support.

American Pain Society (APS)
4700 W. Lake Avenue
Glenview, IL 60025-1485
Phone: 847-375-4715
Fax (Toll-Free): 877-734-8758
Web site: http://www.ampainsoc.org

The mission of this nonprofit membership organization of scientists, clinicians, policy analysts, and others is to advance pain-related research, education, treatment and professional practice. The Web site provides limited publications on pain; some publications can be viewed online and others can be ordered for a fee.

American Society of Clinical Oncology (ASCO)
1900 Duke Street, Suite 200
Alexandria, VA 22314
Toll-Free: 888-651-3038
Phone: 703-299-0150
Fax: 703-299-1044
Web site: http://www.plwc.org

The ASCO is an international medical society representing about 10,000 cancer specialists involved in clinical research and patient care. The ASCO *People Living with Cancer* Web site is a resource for cancer patients, doctors, and researchers and includes patient guides, a glossary of cancer terms, an ASCO member oncologist locator, news and information about different cancers and drug treatments, information about cancer legislation, summaries of government reports, and links to related sites.

Association of Community Cancer Centers (ACCC)
11600 Nebel Street, Suite 201
Rockville, MD 20852-2557
Phone: 301-984-9496
Fax: 301-770-1949
Web site: http://www.accc-cancer.org

This national organization includes over 600 medical centers, hospitals, and cancer programs. This Web site contains a searchable database of cancer centers listed by state as well as information about

oncology drugs (registration is required), and specific cancers.

Cancer Research Institute (CRI)
681 Fifth Avenue
New York, NY 10022
Toll-Free: 800-99-CANCER (800-992-2623)
Phone: 212-688-7515
Fax: 212-832-9376
Web site: http://www.cancerresearch.org

An institute funding cancer research and providing public information on cancer immunology and cancer treatment, the CRI helps patients locate immunotherapy clinical trials, and offers a cancer reference guide and other informational booklets.

City of Hope Pain/Palliative Care Resource Center
1500 East Duarte Road
Duarte, CA 91010
Phone: 626-359-8111, ext. 63829
Fax: 626-301-8941
Web site: http://prc.coh.org

The City of Hope Pain/Palliative Care Resource Center provides information and resources to assist health professionals with improving the quality of pain management. The center offers information on a variety of topics, including pain assessment tools, patient education materials, quality assurance materials, research instruments, and end of life resources. The Web site provides a list of publications and other materials available for order. Over 300 publications are available online. *Some Spanish materials are available.*

International Association for the Study of Pain (IASP)
IASP Secretariat
909 NE 43rd Street, Suite 306
Seattle, WA 98105-6020
Phone: 206-547-6409
Fax: 206-547-1703
Web site: http://www.iasp-pain.org

The IASP, a multidisciplinary, nonprofit professional association, provides information on different topics related to pain on its web site, as well as a list of patient outreach groups and other organizations that provide information on pain and related topics to the general public.

National Cancer Institute (NCI)
NCI Public Inquiries Office
Building 31, Room 10A03
31 Center Drive, MSC 2580
Bethesda, MD 20892-2580
Toll-Free: 800-4-CANCER (800-422-6237)
Web site: http://www.cancer.gov

This government agency provides cancer information through several services (see list below). *Spanish-speaking staff and Spanish materials are available.*

CANCERLIT (Bibliographic Database
Web site:
http://www.cancer.gov/cancerinfo/literature

This searchable site is maintained by the NCI and contains cancer and pain articles published in medical and scientific journals, books, government reports, and articles that were presented at national meetings. A link to the PDQ (CancerNet/NCI database) search engine is provided which allows you to search for clinical trials by state, city, and type of cancer.

CancerTrials
Web site: http://cancertrials.nci.nih.gov

Maintained by the NCI, this site offers information about ongoing cancer clinical trials and explanations of what a trial is and what is involved. A link to the PDQ (CancerNet/NCI database) search engine allows you to search for clinical trials by state, city, and type of cancer.

CancerFax
Fax: 301-402-5874

CancerFax includes information about cancer treatment, screening, prevention, and supportive care. To obtain a contents list, dial the fax number from a fax machine handset and follow the recorded instructions.

CancerNet
Web site:
http://cancer.gov/cancerinformation
Web site (Spanish version):
http://www.cancer.gov/espanol
Web site (online ordering):
https://cissecure.nci.nih.gov/ncipubs/

This comprehensive Web site contains information on diagnosis, treatment, support, resources, literature, clinical trials, prevention and risk factors, and testing. The Physicians Data Query (PDQ) section includes supportive care information—summaries of pain and symptom management for people with cancer. Up to 20 publications can be ordered online. The publications list is searchable. *Some publications are available in Spanish.*

Cancer Information Service (CIS)
Toll-Free: 800-4-CANCER (800-422-6237)
Web site: http://cis.nci.nih.gov

The CIS provides information to consumers and health care professionals. Call CIS for a referral to a pain-control clinic or support group in your area. The Web site contains a wealth of information including pamphlets and brochures on cancer diagnosis, treatment, research, and prevention. *Spanish-speaking staff members are available.*

National Center for Complementary and Alternative Medicine (NCCAM)
Web site: http://altmed.od.nih.gov
NCCAM Clearinghouse
Toll-Free: 888-644-6226

The NCCAM, part of the National Institutes of Health (NIH), facilitates research and evaluation of unconventional medical practices and distributes this information to the public. Their Web site provides information on some complementary and alternative methods promoted as treatments for different diseases.

National Comprehensive Cancer Network (NCCN)
50 Huntingdon Pike, Suite 200
Rockledge, PA 19046
Toll-Free: 800-909-NCCN
Phone: 215-728-4788
Fax: 215-728-3877
Web site: http://www.nccn.org

The NCCN is a nonprofit organization that is an alliance of 19 cancer centers. The American Cancer Society has partnered with NCCN to translate the NCCN Clinical Practice Guidelines into a patient-friendly resource with easy-to-understand information for patients and family members. Treatment guidelines for patients with cancer pain are reprinted in *Appendix B* on page 201. Call the American Cancer Society for the latest guidelines or view them online at either http://www.cancer.org or http://www.nccn.org.

National Library of Medicine (includes MEDLINE)
Web site: http://www.nlm.nih.gov

This National Institutes of Health Web site provides a search engine for health, medical, and scientific literature and research as well as links to other government resources.

PubMed
Web site:
http://www.ncbi.nlm.nih.gov/PubMed

As part of the National Library of Medicine (NLM), this Web site provides access to literature references in Medline and other databases, with links to online journals. The site is searchable by key word.

OncoLink
OncoLink Editorial Board
University of Pennsylvania Cancer Center
3400 Spruce Street-2 Donner
Philadelphia, PA 19104-4283
Web site: http://www.oncolink.com

This Web site provides information on cancer, including educational materials about pain and pain management, support groups, financial questions, and other resources for people with cancer.

Patient and Family Services

American Association of Retired People (AARP)
Dept. # 258390
P.O. Box 40011
Roanoke, VA 24022
Toll-Free: 800-456-2277
Web site: http://www.aarp.org
Web site (for Pharmacy Service):
http://www.aarppharmacy.com

The AARP is a nonprofit membership organization with a commitment to older adults. It provides a variety of services to its members including information on managed care, Medicare, Medicaid, long-term care, and other issues of interest. Membership is open to anyone 50 years old or older. The Web site includes information on a member pharmacy service that offers discounts on drugs used for cancer treatment and pain relief.

Cancer Care, Inc.
275 Seventh Avenue
New York, NY 10001
Toll-Free (Counseling): 800-813-HOPE
(800-813-4637)
Phone: 212-712-8080
Fax: 212-712-8495
Web site: http://www.cancercare.org
Web site (Spanish version): http://www.cancercare.org/EnEspanol/EnEspanolmain.cfm

A nonprofit social service agency, Cancer Care, Inc. provides counseling and guidance to help people with cancer, their families, and friends cope with the impact of cancer. The Web site includes detailed information on specific cancers and cancer treatment, cancer pain, clinical trials, a searchable database of regional and national resources, and links to other sites. The organization also provides videos, free support groups (online, telephone, and face-to-face), workshops, seminars and clinics, a newsletter, and other publications to interested consumers. *Spanish-speaking staff members are available.*

Cancer Survivors Network
American Cancer Society
1599 Clifton Road, NE
Atlanta, GA 30329-4251
Toll-Free: 800-ACS-2345
Web site: http://www.acscsn.org

This network provides an online community that welcomes cancer survivors, friends, and families to share and communicate with others with similar interests and experiences. The program offers a vibrant community of real people supporting one another and sharing personal experiences with cancer. The Web site enables registered members to have live, private chats, to create personal Web pages to share experiences, thoughts, and wisdom, to help people create personal support communities of people who share common concerns and interests, and offers information about resources.

Candlelighters Childhood Cancer Foundation (CCCF)
3910 Warner Street
Kensington, MD 20895
Toll-Free: 800-366-2223
Phone: 301-962-3520
Fax: 301-962-3521
Web site: http://www.candlelighters.org

Candlelighters is an international, nonprofit organization whose mission is to educate, support, serve, and advocate for families of children with cancer, survivors of childhood cancer, and the health care professionals who care for them. CCCF provides a network of parent support groups, an Ombudsman Program offering legal assistance to families of children with cancer and adult survivors of childhood cancer, and publications.

Health Insurance Association of America
555 13th Street, NW, Suite 600 East
Washington, DC 20004
Toll-Free: 800-879-4422
Phone: 202-824-1600

Fax: 202-824-1722

Web site: http://www.hiaa.org

This association represents most United States health insurance companies. The Web site contains insurance guides and general insurance information and an annual directory and survey of hospitals, along with other information.

I Can Cope

American Cancer Society

Toll-Free: 800-ACS-2345

Web site: http://www.cancer.org

This educational program is provided in a supportive environment for adults with cancer and their loved ones. The program offers several courses designed to help participants cope with their cancer experience by increasing their knowledge, positive attitude, and skills. The program is conducted by trained health care professionals in communities throughout the U.S., often with hospital co-sponsorship, as well as in other countries. It offers straightforward cancer information and answers to questions about human anatomy, cancer development, diagnosis, treatment, side effects, new research, communication, emotions, sexuality, self-esteem, and community resources. The program also provides information, encouragement, and practical hints through presentations and class discussions. All classes are free.

Make Today Count

Mid-American Cancer Center

1235 East Cherokee,

Springfield, MO 65804-2263

Toll-Free: 800-432-2273

Phone: 417-885-2273

Fax: 417-888-8761

This is a support organization for people affected by cancer or other life-threatening illness.

Medicare Hotline

Department of Health and Human Services

Toll-Free: 800-MEDICAR

Web site: http://www.medicare.gov

The official U.S. Government site for Medicare provides information on eligibility, enrollment, premiums, coverage, payment and billing, insurance, prescription drugs, and frequently asked questions. Call the toll-free number to receive information about local services.

National Coalition for Cancer Survivorship (NCCS)

1010 Wayne Avenue, Suite 770

Silver Spring, MD 20910

Toll-Free: 877-NCCS-YES

(877-622-7937; general information and publications)

Phone: 301-650-9127

Fax: 301-565-9670

Web site: http://www.canceradvocacy.org/

The NCCS is a survivor-led advocacy organization working in the area of cancer survivorship and support. NCCS seeks to empower survivors by educating all those affected by cancer and speaking out on issues related to quality cancer care. The Web site offers links to online cancer resources, support groups, survivorship programs, a newsletter, and an audio program that teaches skills to help people with cancer meet the challenges of their illness.

National Family Caregivers Association (NFCA)

10400 Connecticut Avenue, Suite 500

Kensington, MD 20895-3944

Toll-Free: 800-896-3650

Phone: 301-942-6430

Fax: 301-942-2302

Web site: http://www.nfcacares.org

This organization is a national, nonprofit, membership association whose mission is to promote caregiving through education and advocacy. NFCA publishes *Take Care!* a newsletter (free for family caregivers) that includes can-do advice, helpful resources, and stories about family caregivers. The NFCA provides referrals to national resources for caregivers and offers a bereavement kit for caregivers. The NFCA Web site provides a report on the status of family caregivers and ten tips for family caregivers.

National Lymphedema Network (NLN)
Latham Square
1611 Telegraph Avenue, Suite 1111
Oakland, CA 94612-2138
Toll-Free (Hotline): 800-541-3259
Phone: 510-208-3200
Fax: 510-208-3110
E-mail: nln@lymphnet.org
Web site: http://www.lymphnet.org

The Web site for this nonprofit agency offers information and education about lymphedema, a referral service to medical and therapeutic treatment centers, and information on locating or establishing local support groups. It publishes a newsletter, which contains articles on lymphedema and related topics, including a resource guide of treatment centers, physicians, therapists, and suppliers. The NLN lists over 100 support groups.

National Self-Help Clearinghouse
Graduate School and University Center of the City University of New York
365 Fifth Avenue, Suite 3300
New York, NY 10016
Phone: 212-817-1822
Fax: 212-817-2990
Web site: http://www.selfhelpweb.org

This nonprofit organization provides access to regional self-help services.

Partnership for Caring: America's Voices for the Dying
1620 Eye Street NW, Suite 202
Washington, DC 20006
Phone: 202-296-8071
Fax: 202-296-8352
Toll-Free: 800-989-9455 (Hotline)
E-mail: pfc@partnershipforcaring.org
Web site: http://www.partnershipforcaring.org

Partnership for Caring: America's Voices for the Dying is a national, nonprofit organization that partners individuals and organizations with the goal of improving how society cares for dying people and their loved ones. Services include: counseling via their 24-hour hotline; publications and videos; information about speaking with family and friends about end-of-life issues; advance directives (living wills and/or medical powers of attorney forms) tailored to each state's legal requirements; and information about state laws on issues such as refusing medical treatment, withdrawing life supports, honoring advance directives, and managing pain.

Pharmaceutical Research and Manufacturers Association of America (PHRMA)
1100 15th Street, NW, Suite 900
Washington, DC 20005
Phone: 202-835-3400
Fax: 202-835-3414
Web site: http://www.phrma.org

PHRMA provides information about member pharmaceutical companies and drugs that are currently available, in use in clinical trials, or under development. The Web site includes a directory of patient assistance programs for prescription drugs and a database of new medications for cancer and other diseases.

Social Security Administration
Department of Health and Human Services
Toll-Free: 800-772-1213
Web site: http://www.ssa.gov

Call the toll-free number to receive information about local services or visit the Web site to learn more about benefits, disability, and other frequently asked-about topics.

TRICARE (formerly CHAMPUS)
Web site: http://www.tricare.osd.mil

TRICARE is part of the military health care system. The Web site offers a link to TRICARE regional offices and a list of phone numbers.

Wellness Community
919 18th Street, NW, Suite 54,
Washington, DC 20006
Toll-Free: 888-793-WELL
Phone: 202-659-9709
Fax: 202-659-9301
E-mail: help@thewellnesscommunity.org
Web site: http://www.thewellnesscommunity.org

The Wellness Community is a nonprofit organization whose mission is to help people with cancer and their families enhance their health and well-being by providing a professional program of emotional support, education, and hope. Support groups are facilitated by licensed psychotherapists. Bereavement support groups are also available. Referrals are provided to their 25 facilities across the nation. The Web site has information about relaxation, talking with children when a parent has cancer, and a study sponsored by the Wellness Community investigating the benefits of a professionally facilitated, online support group for women with breast cancer.

Home and Hospice Care Information

Hospice Association of America (HAA)
228 Seventh Street, SE
Washington, DC 20003
Phone: 202-546-4759
Fax: 202-547-9559
Web site: http://www.hospice-america.org

This nonprofit organization's services include "How to Choose a Hospice"; a hospice locator service; educational programs; and a Web site with information on hospice, HAA programs and materials, and links to related sites.

Hospice Education Institute
3 Unity Square
P.O. Box 98
Machiasport, ME 04655-0098
Toll-Free: 800-331-1620
Phone: 207-255-8800
Fax: 207-255-8008
Web site: http://www.hospiceworld.org

This independent, nationwide, nonprofit organization provides services including: *Hospice Link*, a computerized database and up-to-date directory of all hospice and palliative care programs in the U.S.; general information about principles and practices of good care; and a book and pamphlets on hospice-related topics.

Hospice Foundation of America (HFA)
2001 S. Street, NW, Suite 300
Washington, DC 20009
Toll-Free: 800-854-3402
Phone: 202-638-5419
Fax: 202-638-5312
Web site: http://www.hospicefoundation.org

This organization offers information and materials on hospice care and educational programs. The HFA provides bereavement support and also maintains a current computerized directory of hospices and palliative care programs in the United States. The Web site contains this information along with links to related sites.

Hospice Net
401 Bowling Avenue, Suite 51
Nashville, TN 37205
Web site: http://www.hospicenet.org

A nonprofit organization that works exclusively through its Web site, Hospice Net provides information for patients and caregivers, information about grief and loss, and a hospice locator service.

National Association for Home Care & Hospice (NAHC)
228 Seventh Street, SE
Washington, DC 20003
Phone: 202-547-7424
Web site: http://www.nahc.org

The NAHC provides a state-by-state database of phone numbers for home care and hospice agencies. The NAHC Web site features an online Home Care/Hospice Locator consisting of over 22,000 home care and hospice agencies and information about how to choose a home care agency and/or hospices.

National Hospice and Palliative Care Organization (NHPCO)
1700 Diagonal Road, Suite 300
Alexandria, VA 22314
Toll-Free Helpline: 800-658-8898

Phone: 703-837-1500
Fax: 703-837-1233
Web site: http://www.nhpco.org

This organization is dedicated to providing information about hospice care. The Web site contains related links, a hospice locator database, a newsletter, and other general information.

Visiting Nurse Associations (VNA) of America
99 Summer Street, Suite 1700
Boston, MA 02110
Toll-Free: 888-866-8773
Phone: 617-737-3200
Fax: 617-737-1144
Web site: http://www.vnaa.org

This organization's Web site contains a directory of local VNA agencies, information about choosing a VNA, and answers to questions about home care.

Other Organizations Providing Health and Support Information

Agency for Healthcare Research and Quality (AHRQ)
Publications Clearinghouse
P.O. Box 8547
Silver Springs, MD 20907-8547
Toll-Free: 800-358-9295
Web site: http://www.ahrq.gov

The AHRQ, an office within the U.S. Department of Health and Human Services' Public Health Service, is responsible for supporting research designed to improve the quality of health care, reduce its cost, and broaden access to essential services. One of AHRQ's highest priorities is providing consumers with science-based, easily understandable information that will help them make informed decisions about their own personal health care, including selection of the highest quality health plans and most appropriate health care services.

The American Geriatrics Society Foundation for Health in Aging (FHA)
Toll-Free: 800-563-4916
Web site: http://www.healthinaging.org/public_education/

The FHA's patient education resources were developed in collaboration with the American Geriatrics Society (AGS) and are based on the new major AGS clinical practice guideline for health care providers entitled *The Management of Persistent Pain in Older Persons*. The FHA Web site provides practical and easy-to-use tools to help older adults and their caregivers better manage persistent pain in consultation with their physicians and other health care providers, including: a pain diary and a medication and supplement diary; guides to pain medications, how to assess pain in those with dementia, and information about eldercare at home. Materials may be downloaded and printed from the Web site. Call to obtain hard copies or to place bulk orders.

American Music Therapy Association, Inc. (AMTA)
8455 Colesville Road, Suite 1000
Silver Spring, MD 20910
Phone: 301-589-3300
Fax: 301-589-5175
E-mail: info@musictherapy.org
Web site: http://www.namt.com/

The mission of the AMTA is to advance public awareness of the benefits of music therapy and increase access to quality music therapy services. The Web site includes answers to frequently asked questions, information about music therapy and children and older persons, and related internet resources. Contact AMTA to locate a music therapist in your area.

American Psychological Association (APA)
750 First Street, NE
Washington, DC 20002-4242
Toll-Free: 800-374-2721
Phone: 202-336-5500
Web site: http://www.apa.org

This organization has a Division on Health Psychology that addresses a range of health issues including cancer. The APA provides a hotline patients can use to obtain literature and discuss psychological conditions, and referrals to state psychological associations to locate a psychologist in a specific area. The APA Web site provides a help center with information about psychological issues. *Spanish-speaking staff members are available.*

Joint Commission on Accreditation of Healthcare Organizations (JCAHO)
One Renaissance Boulevard
Oakbrook Terrace, IL 60181
Toll-Free (for filing complaints about a health care organization): 800-994-6610
Phone: 630-792-5000
Fax: 630-792-5005
Web site: http://www.jcaho.org

This is an independent nonprofit organization that evaluates and accredits more than 19,500 health care organizations in the United States, including hospitals, health care networks, and health care organizations that provide home care, long-term care, behavioral health care, and laboratory and ambulatory care services. JCAHO provides information to the public about accreditation status and selecting quality care. Performance reports of accredited organizations and guidelines for choosing a health care facility are available to the public and can be obtained by calling JCAHO or visiting their Web site.

Memorial Sloan-Kettering Cancer Center (MSKCC)
AboutHerbs
Web site:
http://www.mskcc.org/mskcc/html/11570.cfm

Memorial Sloan-Kettering Cancer Center's *AboutHerbs* Web site provides information for consumers about herbs, botanicals, and alternative or unproven cancer therapies, including details about adverse effects, interactions, and potential benefits or problems.

National Association of Social Workers
750 First Street NE, Suite 700
Washington, DC 20002-4241
Toll-Free: 800-638-8799
Phone: 202-408-8600
Fax: 202-336-8340
Web site: http://www.naswdc.org

This organization is concerned with advocacy, work practice standards and ethics, and professional standards for agencies employing social workers. The Web site provides a national register of clinical social workers for local referrals. *Spanish-speaking staff members are available.*

Oncology Nursing Society (ONS)
501 Holiday Drive
Pittsburgh, PA 15220-2749
Phone: 412-921-7373
Fax: 412-921-6565
Web site: http://www.ons.org

This organization is a national membership organization of registered nurses involved in oncology care whose mission is to promote professional standards for oncology nursing, research, and education. Nonmembers can access the ONS web site to find information about cancer treatment, survivorship, and end-of life issues.

Quackwatch
Web site: http://www.quackwatch.com

This Web site provides a guide to fraudulent claims about alternative medicines and questionable health products. The site is searchable by keyword.

World Health Organization (WHO)
WHO Publications Center USA
49 Sheridan Avenue
Albany, NY 12210
Phone: 202-974-3000
Fax: 202-974-3663
Web site: http://www.who.org

The WHO is an agency of the United Nations which promotes technical cooperation for health among nations, carries out programs to control and eradicate disease and to control cancer pain, and strives to improve the quality of human life. The WHO Web site includes data on cancer, a list of publications, and links to related Web sites. *Spanish materials are available.*

•

Glossary

acupuncture: a technique in which very thin needles of varying lengths are inserted into the skin at specific points of the body to treat a variety of conditions, including pain.

acute pain: pain that generally comes on suddenly and lasts a relatively short time.

addiction: a psychological dependence on a medicine; uncontrollable drug craving, seeking, and use. Substance abusers, or addicts, take drugs to satisfy physical, emotional, and psychological needs—not to solve medical problems.

adjuvant analgesic: medicine not originally intended to treat pain, but known to provide pain relief (e.g. antidepressants prescribed to treat nerve pain). See also *analgesic*.

adjuvant therapy: treatment used in addition to the main treatment to increase the chances of curing a disease or prolonging survival.

advance directives: legal documents that tell the doctor and family what a person wants for future medical care, including whether to start or when to stop life-sustaining treatment.

alternative therapy: an unproven therapy used instead of standard (proven) therapy.

analgesic: medicine used to relieve pain.

anesthesia: the loss of feeling or sensation as a result of drugs or gases. General anesthesia causes loss of consciousness ("puts you to sleep"). Local or regional anesthesia numbs only a certain area.

anticonvulsant: medicine used to control seizures; also used to control burning and tingling pain.

antidepressant: medicine used to treat depression; also used as an *adjuvant analgesic* to treat tingling or burning pain from damaged nerves.

antiemetic: medicine used to prevent or relieve nausea and vomiting.

antihistamine: medicine used to control nausea and itching; also used to help people sleep.

biofeedback: treatment method that uses monitoring devices to help people consciously control certain body functions such as heartbeat, blood pressure, and muscle tension. This complementary nondrug method can help control pain.

biopsy: the removal of a sample of tissue to see whether cancer cells are present.

brachytherapy: internal radiation treatment given by placing radioactive material directly into the tumor or close to it; also called interstitial radiation therapy or seed implantation.

breakthrough pain: a flare of pain that occurs when moderate to severe pain is felt for a short time or "breaks through" a regular pain medicine schedule for persistent pain.

catheter: a thin, flexible tube through which fluids enter or leave the body (e.g., a tube to drain urine).

central nervous system: part of the body that includes the brain and spinal cord.

central venous catheter: a special thin, flexible tube placed in a large vein, usually in the chest or neck; it can remain in place for as long as it is needed to deliver medicines or fluids and withdraw blood.

chemotherapy: treatment with drugs to destroy cancer cells.

chronic pain: pain that can range from mild to severe and is present for a long time.

clinical trials: studies of new treatments in patients.

complementary therapy: therapy used in addition to standard therapy. Some complementary therapies may help relieve certain symptoms of cancer, relieve side effects of standard cancer therapy, or improve a patient's sense of well-being. However, complementary therapies do not cure cancer.

corticosteroid: any of a number of naturally occurring or synthetically made substances used to reduce swelling and inflammation. Sometimes used as an anticancer treatment. See also *steroid*.

distraction: a pain-relief method, such as listening to music or using relaxation techniques, in which you turn your attention to something other than the pain.

dose: the amount of medicine taken.

epidural: injection of pain-relief medicine into the space around the sac that encloses the spinal cord.

fine needle aspiration (FNA): in this procedure, a thin needle is used to withdraw (aspirate) samples for examination under a microscope. See also *biopsy*.

frequency: how often medicine is taken.

generic: official name for a medicine, which describes the chemical content of the drug.

home health nurse: a nurse who visits a patient at home to assist with treatments or medications, teaches patients how to care for themselves, and assesses their condition to see if further medical attention is needed.

hospice: a special kind of care for people in the final phase of illness, their families, and caregivers. Hospice care may take place in the patient's home, in a homelike facility, or within hospitals.

hypnosis: a state of restful alertness during which a person enters into a trance-like state, becomes more aware and focused, and is more open to suggestion.

imagery: involves mental exercises that people use to think of pleasant images or scenes, such as waves hitting the beach, to help them relax.

immune system: the complex system by which the body resists infection by microbes such as bacteria or viruses and rejects transplanted tissues or organs. The immune system may also help the body fight some cancers.

incision: a cut made in the skin with a knife.

infusion: a method of giving pain medication into the blood through a vein when slow and/or prolonged delivery of a medicine or fluid is necessary. Unlike an injection, which is given by a syringe, an infusion flows in by gravity or a mechanical pump.

injection: using a syringe and needle to push fluids or medicines into the body; often called a "shot."

intra-arterial: into an artery.

intramuscular (IM): injection into a muscle.

intrathecal (IT): injection into the spinal fluid.

intravenous (IV): a method of administering fluids and medications using a needle or catheter inserted in a vein.

local anesthetic: a medicine that blocks the feeling of pain in a specific location in the body.

long-acting or sustained-release medicines: medicines that work for long periods of time and that are taken at regular intervals during the day and night, such as oral pain-relief medicine that lasts twelve hours. See also *skin patch* and *transdermal*.

lymphedema: a complication that sometimes happens after breast cancer treatments. Swelling in the arm is caused by excess lymph fluid that collects after lymph nodes and vessels are removed by surgery or treated by radiation. This condition can be persistent and may cause some discomfort.

metastasis: the spread of cancer from one part of the body to another.

narcotic: see *opioid*.

nerve block: a process to block pain by injecting pain medicine directly into or around a nerve or into the spine.

neuropathic pain: a dull, burning sensation that can be caused by surgery.

nociceptive pain: pain resulting from damage to body tissue.

nociceptors: pain receptors; thousands of nerve endings located throughout the body.

nonopioid: medicine used for mild to moderate pain.

nonprescription pain medicine: pain-relief medicine that can be bought without a doctor's order; over-the-counter medicine.

nonsteroidal anti-inflammatory drugs (NSAIDs): medicines used to control mild to moderate pain and inflammation. They can be used alone or along with other medicines.

opioid: medicine that acts through the central nervous system to relieve moderate to severe pain.

over-the-counter medicine: pain-relief medicine that can be bought without a doctor's order; nonprescription pain medicine.

pain specialist: a medical professional who is an expert in pain.

pain threshold: the point at which a person becomes aware of pain.

palliative care: treatment that relieves symptoms, such as pain, but is not expected to cure a disease. The main purpose is to improve the patient's quality of life.

patient-controlled analgesia (PCA): a method that allows patients to control the administration of medicines at a rate and dosage that they choose.

persistent pain: pain that is present for long periods of time—in most cases, all day.

phantom limb pain: when a body part is removed during surgery, such as in a mastectomy or amputation, a person may still feel pain or other unpleasant sensations as if they were coming from the missing (phantom) body part.

physical therapy: a treatment used to regain the use of impaired muscles, increase range of motion in joints, relieve pain, and help perform activities of daily living. It involves exercise, electrical stimulation, hydrotherapy, and/or the use of massage, heat, cold, and electrical devices.

port: a small plastic or metal container surgically placed under the skin and attached to a central venous catheter inside the body. Blood and fluids can enter or leave the body through the port.

prostaglandins: substances naturally produced in the body and present in many tissues that perform hormone-like functions.

radiation therapy: treatment with high-energy rays (such as x-rays) to kill or shrink cancer cells. The radiation may come from outside of the body (external radiation) or from radioactive materials placed directly in the tumor (internal or implant radiation). Radiation therapy may be used to reduce the size of a cancer before surgery, to destroy any remaining cancer cells after surgery, or, in some cases, as the main treatment.

rapid-onset opioid: a medicine (opioid) used to relieve pain quickly.

referral pain: pain in one part of the body indicating that a problem exists elsewhere, for example, gallbladder disease is known to produce pain in the right shoulder.

rehabilitation: activities used to help a person adjust, heal, and return to a full, productive life after injury or illness. This may involve physical restoration (such as the use of prostheses, exercises, and physical therapy), counseling, and emotional support.

relaxation techniques: methods used to relieve pain or keep it from getting worse by reducing tension in the muscles.

short-acting medicines: medicines that work quickly and stay in the body for short periods of time, most often used for relief of breakthrough pain. Also called "rescue" medicines.

side effect: an unintended symptom that results from using a medication or is an unwanted effect of treatment, such as hair loss caused by chemotherapy and fatigue caused by radiation therapy.

skin patch: a bandage-like patch that slowly releases medicine that is absorbed through the skin and then into the bloodstream. See also *long-acting medicines* and *transdermal*.

skin stimulation: the use of pressure, friction, temperature change, or chemical substances to stimulate nerve endings in the skin; may lessen or block the feeling of pain.

steroid: a naturally occurring or synthetically made substance used to decrease swelling and inflammation.

subcutaneous infusion: continuous delivery of medicines through a small needle implanted under the skin.

subcutaneous injection (SQ): delivery of medicines through a small needle inserted beneath the skin.

suppository: a small solid substance, usually medication, inserted into an opening of the body, such as the rectum, vagina, or urethra, but *not* the mouth. Once the suppository is inserted in the body, it melts and its medication is absorbed.

tolerance: when the body adjusts to a medicine so that either more or different medicine is needed to relieve pain.

Transcutaneous Electric Nerve Stimulation (TENS): a method of pain relief in which a special device transmits electrical impulses through electrodes to an area of the body that is in pain.

transdermal: a method using a bandage-like skin patch that releases medicine that is absorbed through the skin and into the blood stream. The medicine enters the body slowly and steadily. See also *skin patch*.

transmucosal medicine: medicine in a form that can be absorbed through the lining of the mouth.

Index

E

Ear ringing, 80

Eating difficulties, 17–18, 18, 26
    depression and, 28

Ecotrin, 77

Effexor, *196–197*

Elavil, 87, *198–199*

Elderly persons, cancer pain in
    assessment of, 168–169
    emotional and psychological issues related to, 172
    managing, 169–172

Emphysema, 153

Endep, 87

Endodan, *192–193*

Endometrial biopsy, 14

Endometrial cancer, 110

Endoscopy, 14

Enemas, 146, 148

Epidural infusions, 86, 166

Euthanasia, 181

Ex-Lax, 146

Exercise, 126–127
    fatigue and, *13*

External beam radiation, 107

F

Faces pain rating scale, 68

Family therapy, 36–38

Fatigue, *13*, 20, 23–24, 108, 110

Fear, 28

Fecal impaction, 148, 150

Feelings and attitudes about pain, factors that affect, 25

Feldene, *188–189*

Fenoprofen, *186–187*

Fentanyl citrate, 83, 86, 90, *190–191*

Fentanyl transdermal system, *190–191*

Fiber-containing foods, 146–148, *149*

Fleet, 148

Fluid

    intake, 147–148, *149*
    retention, 80

Fluoxetine hydrochloride, 87, *196–197*

Foods, high-fiber, 146–148, *149*

Fractures, 20, 205

Friend and family support, 30, 36–38

Functional limitations, 17–18, 20, 26

G

Gabapentin, 86, *196–197*

Gastrointestinal (GI) obstruction, 19, 151

Gender and pain, 25

Generic versus brand name drugs, 77

Genpril, *184–185*

Groups, support, 34

Guideline for the Management of Cancer Pain in Adults and Children, 201

H

Haldol, 88, 158, *194–195*

Haloperidol, 158, *194–195*

Haltran, *184–185*

Headaches, 45, 80

Health care professionals
    communicating with, 48–49, 59–61, *153*
    complementary nondrug treatments and, *141*
    mental, 38–40
    notifying about confusion and delirium, *157*
    notifying about constipation, *145*
    notifying about nausea and vomiting, *151*
    notifying about pain, *72*
    notifying about respiratory depression, *154*
    notifying about sedation, *155*
    questions to ask, *60*
    rating pain, 55

Heart rate, increased, 80

Heat applications, 135–136, 167

Hemorrhoids, 91

High-fiber foods, 146–148, *149*

Norpramin, *198–199*
Nortriptyline hydrochloride, *198–199*
Note-taking at health care appointments, 60
Numeric scales for rating pain, 67
Nuprin, 77, 78, *184–185*

O

Olanzapine, 158
Opioids, 44–45, 47, 81–84, *190–193*, 206–208
    addiction to, 44, 97–99, 172–174
    alcohol and, 77
    for breakthrough pain, 95
    central nervous system side effects of,
        153–158
    for children, 165, 166
    confusion and delirium from, 156–158
    constipation from, 144–150
    digestive tract side effects of, 144–153
    for elderly persons, 170–171
    local anesthetics and, 86
    mild, 82–83
    myths about, *98*
    nausea and vomiting from, 150–153
    palliative sedation and, 181
    for patients with a history of substance abuse,
        172–174
    rectal suppositories for delivery of, 91
    respiratory depression from, 153–154
    sedation from, 154–156
    side effects of, 82, 143–158
    strong, 83–84
Oral drug delivery, 89, 105, 165, 171
Oramorph, 83
Orasone, *198–199*
Orudis, *186–187*
Ovarian cancer, 19
Oxazepam, *194–195*
Oxycodone, 83, *192–193*
OxyContin, 83, *192–193*

P

Pain, cancer
    acute, 9, 14–15, 16, 161
    anticipating, 162
    anxiety caused by, 23, 28–30
    assessments, 61–69, 71, 72, 204–205
    bone, 10, 19–20, 111–112, 205, 211
    breakthrough, 10–11, 90, 94–96
    Brief Pain Inventory, 69, *70*
    caregivers' role in helping patients with,
        31–32
    causes of, 13–20
    in children, 160–167
    chronic, 10, 16, 26, 89, *96*
    color scales for rating, 69
    communication about, 46, 48–53, 56–61, 71
    complaining about, 46
    control methods, 3, 11
    counseling and, 32–33
    in culturally diverse groups, 25, 51, 174–177
    decision trees, 203–213
    defining, 8–9
    depression caused by, 24, 26–28
    diagnostic procedures as cause of, 13–15
    in elderly persons, 168–172
    faces scale for rating, 68
    factors that influence, 12–13
    feelings about, 25–30
    focusing on, 46
    functional limitations caused by, 17–18, 20, 26
    gastrointestinal (GI) obstruction, 19
    identifying and expressing, 3
    immobility as cause of, 20
    impact of, 1–3, 23–24
    as indication of course of illness, 45
    individual reactions to, 26
    infections as cause of, 205
    intracranial, 19
    language of, 56–58
    logs, 71–72, *73*, 101–102, *103*

management guidelines, 201
measuring, 61–69
medication side effects, 47–48, *184–199*
myths and misconceptions about, 44–48
nerve damage and, 20
neuropathic, 12
nociceptive, 11
as not unavoidable, 45
numeric scales for rating, 67
palliative therapy for, 106–112
in patients with advanced disease, 177–181
in patients with history of substance abuse,
  172–174
phantom limb, 17
quality of life and, 23–24
questions to ask health care team about, *60*
rating scales, 67–69
recurrence after treatment, 72
relationship impact of, 30–32
subjective nature of, 51–52
in terminally ill patients, 178–181
"toughing out," 47
treatment plans, 69, 71
treatments as cause of, 15–18
tumor-related, 19–20
types of, 9–12
undertreatment of, 2
word scales for rating, 68
words for describing, 56–58
Palliative therapy
  bisphosphonate, 111
  chemotherapy, 109–110
  hormonal, 110
  in patients with advanced disease, 177–178
  radiation, 106–109
  sedation, 180–181
  surgical, 111–112
Pamelor, *198–199*
Paroxetine hydrochloride, 87, *196–197*
Pastoral counselors, *39*
Patient-controlled analgesia (PCA), 93

Paxil, 87, *196–197*
Percocet, *192–193*
Percodan, *192–193*
Peri-Colace, 146
Peripheral nerve blocks, 116
Peripherally inserted central catheters, 91
Permanent nerve blocks, 114–115
Persistent pain, 10–11
Pertofrane, *198–199*
Phantom limb pain, 17
Phenytoin, 86
Physical dependence on medications, 99
Physical examinations, 62–63
Piroxicam, *188–189*
Pneumonia, 153
Prayer, 122, 138–139
Prednisone, 87, *198–199*
Preparation for pain assessments, 63–66
Pressure treatments, 137
Prochlorperazine, 152
Progressive muscle relaxation, 133
Prostaglandins, 77
Prostate cancer, 110
Prozac, 87, *196–197*
Psychiatric/mental health nurses, *39*
Psychiatrists, *39*
Psychodynamic therapy, 36
Psychological assessments, 63
Psychological dependence and addiction, 44,
  97–99, 172–174
Psychologists, *39*
Psychosocial support services, 32–33
  choosing a counselor for, 38–40
  determining need for, 40–41
  for elderly patients, 172
  family therapy, 36–38
  group, 34
  individual, 35–36
  insurance coverage for, 42
  self-help, 35
Psychotherapy, 35–36, 122, 132–133, 166

Q
Quality of life and pain, 23–24

R
Radiation therapy, 101, 106–108, *109*, 151
  pain due to, 9, 18, 45, 161
  palliative, 106–108, *109*
  side effects, 18, 108
Radiopharmaceuticals, 107
Reactions to pain, 26
Rectal suppositories, 91, 171
Reglan, 152
Relationships, impact of pain on, 30–32
Relaxation, 122, 131, 133–135, 166
Religion. *See* Prayer; Spirituality
Respiratory depression, 153–154
Rhizotomy, 118
Rhythmic massage, 133
Ringing in the ears, 80
Rofecoxib, 78, *188–189*
Ropivacaine, 86
Roxicodone, *192–193*
Roxiprin, *192–193*
Rufen, *184–185*

S
Salflex, *184–185*
Salsalate, *184–185*
Sedation, 154–156
  of children, 164
  palliative, 180–181
Selective serotonin reuptake inhibitors (SSRIs), *85, 87, 196–197*
Self-help groups, 35
Senna, 146
Senokot, 146
Serax, *194–195*
Sertraline, 87
Serzone, *196–197*

Sexual function, 110
Shortness of breath, 108
Side effects
  acetaminophen, 81
  central nervous system, 153–158
  chemotherapy, 17–18, 45, 81, 110, 130, 132, 151
  depression as, 28
  digestive tract, 144–153
  nerve block, 113–114, 115
  nonsteroidal anti-inflammatory drug (NSAID), 79–80
  opioid, 82, 143–158
  pain medication, 47–48, *85, 184–199*, 212
  radiation therapy, 18–19, 108–109
  spinal opioid infusion, 117–118
  surgery, 16–17
Sinequan, 87, *196–197*
Skin patches, 90
Skin stimulation, 121, 135–138
Sleep, 23–24, 26, 131
  depression and, 28
  fatigue and, *13*
  and sedation caused by opioids, 154–156
Slow rhythmic breathing, 133–135
Social activities, effect of pain on, 24
Social workers, *39*
Spinal opioid infusion, 117–118
Spinal taps, 15, 164
Spirituality, 26, 138–139
Stomach bleeding, 79
Stomas, 91
Stool softeners, 146–147
Stress, 23, 128–129, 130, 131
Strong opioids, 83–84
Subcutaneous injection, 92, 171
Subjective nature of pain, 51–52
Sublingual drug delivery, 90
Substance abuse, cancer patients with a history of, 172–174

We Care about Your Opinions.

Please take a moment to complete this survey and fax it to *Books/Product Marketing Specialist* at **404-325-9341**, or email your comments and suggestions to us at **trade.sales@cancer.org**. *Thank you!*

PLEASE PRINT.

First Name _____

Last Name _____

Address _____

City _____ State _____ Zip _____

Email _____

1. Gender: ☐ Female ☐ Male

2. Age: ☐ 20–39 ☐ 40–59 ☐ 60+

3. How many health books have you bought or read in last 12 months? _____

4. How did you find out about this book? (Please choose one.)
   ☐ Recommendation ☐ Store Display ☐ Online
   ☐ Advertisement ☐ Catalog/Mailing ☐ TV/Radio

5. Did this book meet your needs? _____

_____

6. What attracts you most to a book? (Please rank 1–4 in order of preference; 1 being most important.)
   ____ Title ____ Content ____ Cover Design ____ Author

7. If you would you like more information about other books published by the American Cancer Society, please tell us how you prefer to be contacted:
   ☐ Email ☐ Mail